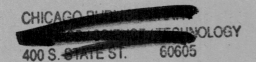

GUNSHOT WOUNDS
Pathophysiology and Management

Kenneth G. Swan, MD
Professor of Surgery
College of Medicine and Dentistry of New Jersey
New Jersey Medical School

Roy C. Swan, MD
Joseph C. Hinsey Professor of Anatomy
Cornell University Medical College

PSG Publishing Company, Inc.
Littleton, Massachusetts

Library of Congress Cataloging in Publication Data

Swan, Kenneth G
  Gunshot wounds.

  Includes bibliographical references and index.
    1. Gunshot wounds. I. Swan, Roy C., joint author.
II. Title. [DNLM: 1. Wounds, Gunshot. WO807 S972g]
RD96.3.S93   617'.145   79-16118
ISBN 0-88416-196-X

Printed in the United States of America.

International Standard Book Number: 0-88416-196-X

Library of Congress Catalog Card Number: 79-16118

To our father, Roy C. Swan, Sr., whose vocation and avocations
generated in him a passion for the safe handling of firearms.

Pharmacology is an ever-changing science. As new research and clinical experience broaden our knowledge, changes in treatment and drug therapy are required. The editors and the publisher of this work have made every effort to ensure that the treatment and drug dosage schedules herein are accurate and in accord with the standards accepted at the time of publication. Readers are advised, however, to check the product information sheet included in the package of each drug they plan to administer to be certain that changes have not been made in the recommended dose or in the indications and contraindications for administration. This recommendation is of particular importance in regard to new or infrequently used drugs.

CONTENTS

FOREWORD

This book is a timely documentation of the pathophysiology and management of gunshot wounds as seen in the clinical setting. It serves as a form of increasing recognition of what previously has been termed "the neglected disease of modern society." Trauma is a surgical illness that is continuously increasing in our society. It is now the leading cause of death in the first three decades of life as well as the third leading cause of death in all ages. In spite of these appalling statistics, only recently have clinical and research data been organized in an attempt to improve the care of the injured patient.

Gunshot Wounds indicates that each year in the United States nearly 30,000 people are fatally wounded by firearms. This is more than half the number of people (50,000) killed in the United States each year in motor vehicle accidents. Interestingly, the incidence of fatal wounds by firearms is increasing, as is mortality from trauma of all kinds. It is equally true, however, that the morbidity and mortality rates for patients having sustained trauma are improving annually. As pointed out here, a combination of several factors contributes to the continuing increase in survival of patients sustaining all forms of trauma. Biologic support of the injured patient, which is a subtle improvement, has served as a major factor in the salvage of the traumatized patient. Well-organized, detailed, and prompt management of patients having sustained injury (including gunshot wounds) is also showing a significant impact on survival as well as decreasing the morbidity from these injuries.

As the authors point out, the current monograph is a survey of a large clinical experience with injured patients, with appropriate review of management used in specific injuries. Controversial areas of management are generally indicated throughout the text but the overall organization, and current state-of-the-art approach is well presented. Certainly, the work on ballistics is unique and normally has not been presented in the concentrated and organized fashion seen in this book.

Work such as this will surely stimulate critical appraisal. It should also create an awareness of the magnitude of the problem of trauma. This will ultimately result in better care of the injured patient.

G. Tom Shires, MD
Professor and Chairman
Cornell University Medical College
and The New York Hospital

PREFACE

This book is intended for the general surgeon, the specialist in emergency medicine, and the military surgeon-to-be, all of whom will find interest in an overview of the management of trauma caused by moderate- to high-velocity missiles. The term *gunshot wound* as used historically, has lost some of its appropriateness today. Comparable wounds caused by missiles can result from a variety of sources other than guns. In civilian life, causative agents range from rotary lawn mowers to industrial explosions; in warfare, from hand grenades to bomb blasts. Regardless of etiology, the principals of the management of such wounds are similar.

While intended for the generalist, the discussion of management extends well into the provinces of the surgical specialties, not with the implication that the generalist should acquire such special expertise, but to give him a sense of the urgency for and complexity, as well as capability, of special care, and a frame of reference for improvisation when such help is unavailable.

The first three chapters address general principles. From there, patient wound management is discussed in terms relevant to the region wounded. In general, this discussion focuses on regional anatomy, but occasionally the need arises to address a category of wounds in terms of the related surgical discipline. For example, the principles of nerve repair are discussed in the chapter on the neck, but these principles are also applicable to facial nerve repair.

This book is a summary of the state of the art as we see it today, now that the Vietnam experience has been digested and the increasing trauma of civilian life is demanding more precise and efficient organization of emergency care of the injured. This state of the art has been arrived at in recent decades by untold numbers of trials, innovations, and resultant new concepts in the medical specialties, not by any single new philosophy revolutionizing the management of gunshot wounds, such as preceded the classic treatises on this subject by Paré, Hunter, and others in previous centuries.

What is the prospect for new concepts in the management of gunshot wounds? What directions will they take? We hope that this book will be grossly out of date in 10 to 15 years, not through any expectation that the incidence of such trauma will be less, but due to new concepts and techniques in the restoration of blood circulation, in regional reconstruction, and in regeneration of muscle, bone, blood vessel, and nerve tissue and of even more complex tissues and organs. We anticipate it will also be greatly outdated in 10 to 15 years by better organization and training in civilian triage and emergency care of the victim of trauma. Meanwhile, we expect this book will narrow the gap between the state of the art today and the general quality of practice in the care of gunshot wounds.

ACKNOWLEDGMENTS

The authors gratefully acknowledge the help and contributions of the following people:

Brig Gen Thomas J. Whelan (MC, USA [Ret]) inspired and supported a special assignment in Vietnam in 1970 to document, in color photography, the surgical management of combat casualties. Col Robert J.T. Joy (MC, USA, former Director of the Walter Reed Army Institute of Research) provided command emphasis and logistic support to this assignment. The assignment resulted in the Vietnam Trauma Slide Collection consisting of over 200 cases and 6500 transparencies, some of which are included in this book. Col Mahlon V.R. Freeman (MC, USA [Ret], former Associate Director of Medical Education of the Armed Forces Institute of Pathology) provided editorial skills for the processing of the Vietnam Trauma Slide Collection. Benjamin F. Rush, Jr., MD (Johnson and Johnson Professor and Chairman of the Department of Surgery of the College of Medicine and Dentistry of New Jersey–New Jersey Medical School), gave valuable support and criticism. Col Christine E. Haycock (MC, USAR, Associate Professor of Surgery, CMDNJ–NJ Medical School) inspired basic ballistic studies of the comparative effects of modern weapons of war upon simulated human tissue. This resulted in a shared exhibit with the author, "Gunshot Wounds," to the American College of Surgeons, 1975–1979. Martin G. Levine, PhD (Director of Biomedical Communications, CMDNJ–NJ Medical School) provided outstanding technical support of pictorial and tabular data found within this text. Ms Donna G. Di Salvo (Executive Secretary, Department of Surgery, CMDNJ–NJ Medical School) typed and edited the manuscript with devotion above and beyond the call of duty. Finally, the authors acknowledge the understanding and patience of their wives, Betsy and Beatrice.

The following photographs are printed with the courtesy of U.S. Army-Vietnam Surgical Trauma Collection, Armed Forces Institute of Pathology, Washington, D.C.: Figures 4-1–4-3, 4-10, 5-1–5-6, 6-1–6-9, 6-11–6-24, 7-1–7-11, 8-1–8-24, 9-1–9-4, 9-22–9-30, 9-34 and 9-35.

INTRODUCTION

Second only to motor vehicles as instruments of death, firearms will
kill more than 28,000 Americans this year.*

Currently, in the United States, nearly 30,0C0 people are fatally
wounded by firearms annually.[1] This number is more than half of the
total United States military fatalities in the 12 years (1961–1973)[2] of the
Vietnam War (57,000) and more than half the number of people killed
in the United States each year in motor-vehicle accidents (50,000).[3] Not
only is the incidence of fatal wounds by firearms increasing in this
country, but more extensive and destructive wounds are being encountered as firearms capable of propelling higher-velocity missiles
are being introduced into crime and sporting activities. When nonfatal
and fatal wounds by firearms are added (the ratio is 10 to 1, at least),
along with the incidence of wounds by high-velocity missiles from
sources other than firearms (e.g., terrorist bomb blasts, industrial
explosions, etc.), a major threat to health and survival in the United
States is defined.

In parallel with these trends is ·the developing competence of
American medicine to correct and compensate for very destructive
lesions of trauma. The care of combat-injured United States troops
in Vietnam was exemplary. The killed-in-action/wounded-in-action
ratio (KIA/WIA) was the highest recorded in the history of warfare
(1/6.5) and exceeded that for the more recent Yom Kippur War in
1973.[2] This amazing statistic reflects a combination of advanced
helicopter air-ambulance evacuation capability and superbly staffed,
secure, fixed installations for the care of the wounded.

Today, major lesions of the pump and the conduits in the circulatory system can be repaired or replaced. Major incursions upon
respiration can be reversed. Major and proximal interruptions in
peripheral neural transmission can be repaired. Disastrous threats to
central neural function can be minimized. Extensive skeletal damage
can be repaired or replaced by prostheses. Replantation of amputated
extremities is currently successful in almost three-fourths of such
patients.[4] Extensive epithelial defects can be replaced by grafts. And
looking to the future, the technology of cell culture[5] encourages the
expectation for more practical reconstruction of epithelium and the
reconstitution of muscle, bone, and eventually other tissues.

Currently, there exists a wide gulf between this major social
threat—wounds by high-velocity missiles—and the potential for
human repair by tertiary medical care. Most medical professionals and

*Editorial in *J Trauma,* June, 1976.

paraprofessionals are unlikely to encounter gunshot wounds frequently enough to bridge efficiently and effectively the gulf between wounding and definitive care. The encounter usually provides no time for review and research by the primary physician. The hard-won lessons of military medicine are dissipated in peacetime. Opportunities for salvage are wasted.

This short book can serve the continuing education of the generalist, the paraprofessional, the military surgeon-to-be, and the specialist in emergency medicine. If in the professional lifetime of any such individuals, it guides the appropriate management between wounding and definitive care, it will be worth the two to three evenings required for its reading.

The principles outlined in the succeeding chapters are, we believe, consistent with the principles of modern, first-class surgery. Their evolution is based upon the experience of military surgeons over half a millennium. They are personally reinforced by the experience of one of the authors (K.G.S.) who served as a United States Army surgeon in Vietnam during the years 1968 through 1970, as a civilian consultant to the Department of Surgery of the University of Saigon Medical School in Vietnam in 1975, and since then, as director of surgery in the city hospital within the center of a large urban ghetto.

REFERENCES

1. Baker, S.P. 28,000 gun deaths a year: what is our role? *J Trauma.* 16:510–511, 1976.

2. The World Almanac and Book of Facts, 1979. New York: Newspaper Enterprise Assoc. Inc., 1979, p. 333.

3. *The New York Times,* 15 February 1979, p. 22.

4. Jablon, M., and Kleinert, H.E. An overview of replantation results of 347 replants in 245 patients since 1970. *J Trauma.* (In press) Presented at the 39th Annual Meeting of the American Association for the Surgery of Trauma. Chicago, September 13–15, 1979.

5. Green, H. Studies on a complex epithelial cell in culture. *Harvey Lectures* (In press).

1 History

Gunshot wounds are now becoming almost a distinct branch of surgery.*

The introduction of firearms in Europe in the fourteenth century presented surgeons with what they considered a distinctly new problem, the gunshot wound. Prior experience with penetrating wounds had been limited to those resulting from more cleanly cutting, much lower velocity missiles and weapons in which the path and presence of the penetrating object were usually obvious and the contamination of the wound usually less. Centuries were to pass before surgeons understood the cause and nature of the inflammation, the mechanisms of contamination of wounds, the consequences of removing or not removing the missile, and the relation between velocity of impact and extent of damage. It is true that by the early twentieth century, we had gained the basic understanding of inflammation, infection, terminal

---

*Hunter, J. *A Treatise on the Blood, Inflammation and Gunshot Wounds.* London: G. Nicol, 1794.

1

ballistics, and cavitation, and had general control of the problems through concepts of first aid, hemostasis, debridement, antisepsis, antibiotics, and reconstructive surgery. However, the field is not static, and we must now ask whether our understanding of a high-velocity missile wound is keeping pace with the development of firearms of very high velocity.

The history of the treatment of gunshot wounds is inseparably tied to the history of the development of firearms, the history of their military use, and the history of general and special surgery. The causal chain is by no means as simple as might be inferred from the following brief account. As is usually the case in the development of understanding and treatment of other forms of trauma, interest and innovation in the treatment of gunshot wounds have always peaked in wartime, and the prominent innovations and writings on the subject have come through the experience of military surgeons. The concepts and practices thus tend to reflect that which was applicable to numerous casualties on or near the battlefield, rather than that which the experience and understanding of these surgeons might have allowed them to apply to an occasional case in a civilian setting.

Most impressive about gunshot wounds of the fifteenth and early sixteenth centuries was their relatively greater inflammation and suppuration as compared to previously encountered penetrating wounds. Today, we attribute this to the relatively greater amount of contaminated foreign matter propelled through or drawn into the wound. In those days, however, the belief became prevalent that bullets or gunpowder burned or poisoned tissue. Heroic methods were directed at removing the bullet and the poison. Sounds and forceps for locating and removing the bullet were applied early and determinedly. To facilitate their use, the wound was dilated by instruments, swelling packs, or incisions. To withdraw the poison from the wound, foreign material, often horse hair, was drawn through the wound, and various oils, often hot, and even boiling, were poured into the wound. The copious suppuration thus induced was applauded as combating the poison and heralding a favorable outcome. Amputation for extensive tissue destruction by gangrene was recommended, but there was much disagreement as to whether the incision should be through gangrenous or healthy tissue. The ancient Greeks had recommended the latter, but the fear of hemorrhage tended to restrict the surgeons of the Renaissance to incisions through the gangrenous tissue, or at its margin with viable tissue. Hemorrhage from the wound was recognized as an unlikely early, but frequent secondary, complication. The principle of the tourniquet had not yet been introduced, nor the physiologic basis for its application yet developed. The anatomic and physiologic understanding for effective acupressure did not generally exist. Ligation, as recommended by the ancient physicians, had been discarded.

Cautery by hot irons or boiling oil was used to achieve hemostasis in the wound or amputation stump.

These principles were set forth in the earliest publications on the treatment of gunshot wounds by the itinerant, poorly educated, and highly specialized "wound surgeons" of northern Europe, notably Pfolspeundt (1447), Brunschwig (1497), and von Gerssdorf (1517), as well as by the classically educated, more generalized surgeons of Italy, such as da Vigo (1514).[1]

By the mid-sixteenth century, largely in the writings of Maggi in Italy (1542) and Paré in France (1545), came recognition that wounded tissue was crushed rather than poisoned or burned, that the prevailing heroic methods directed at extracting poison and promoting suppuration were more harmful than beneficial, and that the body had a greater capacity for natural healing of wounds than previously thought. Both Maggi and Paré discarded cauterization of the wound.

Celsus, Galen, and Avicenna had, in ancient and medieval times, recommended control of hemorrhage by mass ligation. The surgeons of the Renaissance, with the exception of Vesalius, had rejected such ligation as too time-consuming and clumsy. In the light of Vesalius' *DeFabrica Humani Corporis* and with the development of improved surgical instrumentation, Ambroise Paré (1510–1590), the greatest surgeon of his time, reintroduced ligation. With better hemostasis, he was then able to espouse the principle that in amputation, the incision should be through proximal healthy tissue.

Paré, followed by Paracelsus in the seventeenth century, John Hunter in the eighteenth century, and Larrey in the nineteenth century, each of whom published classic contributions to the nature and treatment of gunshot wounds, kept alive the insight of Hugh de Lucca, Théodoric, and Mondeville, the great medieval physicians, into the natural capacity of wounded tissue for healing and the feasibility of primary closure. Each opposed prevailing practices of intervention which, from the perspective of modern microbiology, would today be considered harmful.

Until the mid-nineteenth century, the treatment of gunshot wounds was largely restricted to wounds of the extremities and to superficial wounds of the trunk, head, and neck. Wounds involving the body cavities and joints were regarded as inevitably fatal, although trephination was performed for increased intracranial pressure caused by hemorrhage or suppuration, and attempts were made to elevate the depressed inner table of the calvarium and remove cranial bone splinters.[2]

The treatment of gunshot wounds in the eighteenth century was characterized by a bolder and earlier use of amputation, a greater latitude in the choice of sites for such, and the development of an alternative—exarticulation. Before then, amputation was usually approached with dread, resorted to late in the face of progressive gangrene, and used when an otherwise fatal outcome was inevitable. In addition, incisions to achieve flap closure of the stump came into use. Following the introduction of the tourniquet by Morel in 1674, ligation became more precise and less massive. Better prostheses were developed. These factors, coupled with considerations of expedience in the face of large numbers of battlefield casualties and limited facilities for transport and hospitalization, contributed to a less discriminative and earlier resort to amputation. Along with this there developed enthusiasm for wide, deep, and multiple incisions of the wound in order to remove the bullet and promote drainage. Excess trephination and exposure to the dura for even minor head wounds prevailed. In reaction to these trends came Hunter's clear, conservative, and influential publication on inflammation and gunshot wounds in 1794, based on his three years as a military surgeon in Portugal (1761–1763).[3] Hunter, whom Billroth credited with being the father of modern (i.e., nineteenth-century) English and German surgery, limited the indications for surgery to (1) hemorrhage and the need for ligation, (2) the removal of bony fragments, (3) the removal of a dangerous foreign body, (4) the replacement of eviscerated organs, and (5) relief of pressure impairing the function of a vital organ.

The early nineteenth century saw a resurgence in the use of amputation for gunshot wounds of the extremities. In the context of the large battles and massive casualties of the Napoleonic wars, primary amputation within a few hours of the injury, became the most important surgical operation. Larrey, Napoleon's Surgeon General, reported performing 200 amputations in one day at the battle of Borodino (1812).[4] Comparably engaged were British surgeons under Guthrie, Larrey's counterpart in the Peninsular wars and at Waterloo.[5] Larrey and Guthrie, in the face of limited transport and septic conditions in rear hospitals, advised prompt amputation on or near the battlefield, for all compound fractures of the extremities and *all* gunshot wounds of the thigh. Guthrie[6] recognized the need for early arterial ligation, distally as well as proximally, even in the absence of hemorrhage.

Although surgeons still approached wounds of the thorax with great trepidation, the beginning of the nineteenth century brought systematic consideration of when to close such wounds and when to drain blood and exudate. Even da Vigo, in 1514, had discussed the problem in connection with a case report of a gunshot wound penetrating the thoracic wall. He apparently had some insight into the danger to respiration of blood accumulating in the pleural cavity, as had Paré.[7] Tension pneumothorax had been explained in 1767 by Hewsom, a colleague of Hunter. However, general understanding of respiratory mechanics and the principle of closed drainage were not to play parts in surgery until late in World War I.

Terminal ballistics and tissue damage as a function of distance along the bullet track came under more explicit consideration during the nineteenth century. There also was more concern for the general health and nutrition of the wounded patient. Tetanus was variously attributed to drying or chilling of wounded nerves or tendons. Hospital gangrene became recognized as a contagious complication of wound suppuration. Somewhat effective systemic measures for managing increased intracranial pressure in head wounds came into use, and more conservative and specific indications for trephination were defined. Wounds of the abdominal cavity remained forbidden territory to surgical intervention.

The latter half of the nineteenth century brought in the new science of bacteriology under Pasteur and Koch. Soon followed the revolution in surgery occasioned by Lister's recognition that wounds were infected by microorganisms, and his introduction of antiseptic surgery. Along with this came success in intraabdominal surgery and effective management of intraabdominal gunshot wounds. Klebs systematically studied the bacteriology of gunshot wounds and showed that a filtrate of wound exudate was not infectious. By World War I, surgeons had gained substantial control over wound infections.

The increase in muzzle velocity, achieved by the replacement of black powder by smokeless powder, and the introduction of rifled gun barrels brought a new phenomenon into gunshot wounds—a more destructive feature at first suspected to be due to "explosive" bullets. In 1898, Woodruff[8] explained this new destructiveness as secondary to cavitation, a phenomenon that has come under intensive analysis and grown in importance within the past 30 years.

Military surgical experience gained from the management of combat casualities sustained by U.S. troops during World War II indicated that ligation of major arterial injuries was no longer the treatment of choice, and that whenever possible, reconstruction of the injured vessel was preferable. During the Korean War, this trend toward a more definitive treatment of vascular trauma was augmented by the introduction of the autologous saphenous vein interposition grafting as an additional technique for major arterial reconstruction attending the management of vascular trauma secondary to war wounds.[9] As a result of the recent Vietnam War, U.S. military surgeons recognized the need for an additional modification of existing protocols regarding the management of vascular trauma, namely, that injury to concomitant veins should be treated with primary repair for two reasons: (1) the previously accepted treatment, ligation, resulted in a marked reduction in associated arterial inflow and thus jeopardized the patency of the arterial repair; (2) the resultant decrease in arterial inflow also jeopardized the viability of the limb which often had sustained multiple injuries in addition to the major vascular damage.[10]

In the twentieth century, the term *gunshot wound,* although still in wide use, can no longer be used with any degree of precision. The exponential increases in velocity, power, and destructiveness of firearms, especially those for military use, have brought the management of wounds due to modern weapons closer to the concepts of the management of the other general types of trauma such as crush, blast, burn, radiation, and other forms of extensive disruption and destruction of tissue. The challenge of the twentieth century, with respect to the management of such wounds, has become one of dealing with the systemic problems threatening survival in the first few hours and the later problems of reconstruction and rehabilitation. The nature of wounds from firearms in this century is probably as different from those of the last as were the wounds from firearms in the fifteenth century from sword and arrow wounds. Yet, the historic threads between the concepts of the nature and management of wounds from firearms over the past six centuries are strong.

REFERENCES

1. Billroth, C.A.T. Historical studies on the nature and treatment of gunshot wounds from the fifteenth century to the present time. Translated by C.P. Rhoads. *Yale J Biol Med.* 4:16–36, 119–148, 225–257, 1931–1932.

2. Garrison, F.A. *Introduction to the History of Medicine.* 4th Ed. Philadelphia: W.B. Saunders Co., 1929.

3. Hunter, J. *A Treatise on the Blood, Inflammation and Gunshot Wounds.* London: G. Nicol, 1794.

4. Dibble, J.H. *Napoleon's Surgeon General.* London: Heinemann, 1970.

5. Blanco, R.L. *Wellington's Surgeon: Sir James McGrigor.* Durham, N.C.: Duke University Press, 1974.

6. Guthrie, G.J. *On Gunshot Wounds of the Extremities Requiring the Different Operations of Amputations with Their After Treatment.* London: Longman, 1815.

7. Churchill, E.D. *Surgeon to Soldiers.* Philadelphia: J.B. Lippincott, Co., 1972, pp. 443–455.

8. Woodruff, C.E. The causes of the explosive effect of modern small caliber bullets, *NY Med J.* 67:593–601, 1898.

9. Rich, N.M., and Spencer, F.C. *Vascular Trauma.* Philadelphia: W.B. Saunders Co., 1978.

10. Swan, K.G. (Ed.). *Venous Surgery in the Lower Extremities.* St Louis, Mo.: Warren H. Green, 1975.

2 Wound Ballistics

Then came reports of frightful destruction of tissue, just as though the bullet had exploded.*

Ballistics is the science of the motion of a projectile during its travel through the barrel of a firearm, during its subsequent trajectory through air, and during its final complicated motion after striking the target. Wound ballistics is a special case of the latter—when the target is animal tissue.[1-4] Principles of wound ballistics are crucial to the evaluation of gunshot wounds and their treatment. This is becoming increasingly apparent, as the development of weaponry in recent decades has moved toward progressively smaller projectiles and increasingly higher velocities. This developmental trend will undoubtedly continue, at least into the foreseeable future.

A low-velocity (< 1000 ft/sec, or < 305 m/sec), 22-caliber† (5.6-mm-

---

*Woodruff, C.E. The causes of the explosive effects of modern small caliber bullets. *NY Med J.* 67:593–601, 1898.

†Caliber is the diameter of a bullet or rifle bore in hundredths (2 digit) or thousandths (3 digit) of an inch.

diameter bullet) pistol wound of soft tissue, such as the calf, will exhibit an entrance and an exit wound even less than the diameter of the bullet and a track of tissue damage not much greater in diameter (Figure 2-1A). Usually, this wound will not require debridement. A higher-velocity (> 3000 ft/sec, or > 914 m/sec) gunshot wound, such as that resulting from a bullet of the same caliber from the current U.S. military rifle (M-16 A1) or comparable military or sporting rifle, may exhibit a similar entrance, but the exit may vary from the same to many times the diameter of the bullet (Figure 2-1E,F). Conversely, there may be no exit (Figure 2-1C), or an enormous exit (Figure 2-1E), depending upon the bullet and the type of tissues encountered.[4] The track of this high-velocity, rapidly decelerating, and deforming projectile may be surrounded by tissue destruction extending up to several centimeters radially from the track, due to a momentary intense compression and subsequent stretching of surrounding tissue to 10 to 30 times its normal dimensions (Figure 2-1B). Projectiles fired at velocities approaching and exceeding 5000 ft/sec, or 1524 m/sec from weapons now under development and destined to be used in future combat, and inevitably to come into the hands of hunters and felons, will predictably cause explosive and extensive damage up to several centimeters in all directions from the point of impact and have no exit (Figure 2-1H). Wounds from such projectiles will present major problems in surgical reconstruction. Thus, the characteristics of gunshot wounds range from those from low-velocity projectiles fired from common handguns, in which the resultant tissue damage may not be much more extensive than that caused by a slowly penetrating, sharp rod of similar diameter, to those from very-high-velocity, small-caliber projectiles, in which a very large, but relatively shallow, mass of damaged tissue extends several centimeters in all directions from the point of impact. Such might be imagined from a small, subcutaneously implanted, explosive charge, or from a large, blunt object striking with extreme force.

Two principles are basic to an understanding of the form and extent of tissue damage in gunshot wounds. The first concerns the interrelation of factors determining the dissipation of the kinetic energy of a projectile in tissues.[5] The second concerns the phenomenon of cavitation in the wound.

DISSIPATION OF KINETIC ENERGY

As in the case of ionizing particle radiation damage to tissue, the extent and degree of damage in wounds is proportional to the amount

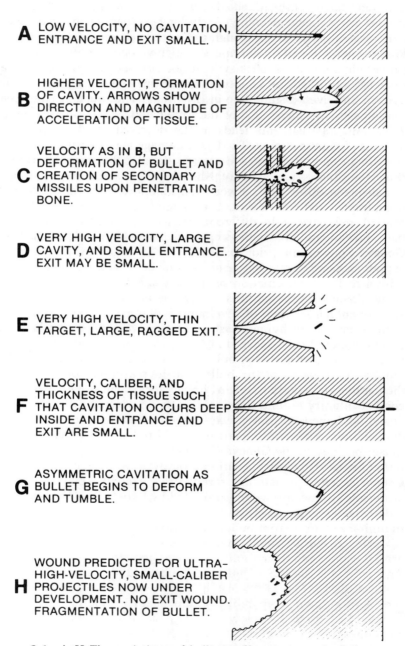

A LOW VELOCITY, NO CAVITATION, ENTRANCE AND EXIT SMALL.

B HIGHER VELOCITY, FORMATION OF CAVITY. ARROWS SHOW DIRECTION AND MAGNITUDE OF ACCELERATION OF TISSUE.

C VELOCITY AS IN **B**, BUT DEFORMATION OF BULLET AND CREATION OF SECONDARY MISSILES UPON PENETRATING BONE.

D VERY HIGH VELOCITY, LARGE CAVITY, AND SMALL ENTRANCE. EXIT MAY BE SMALL.

E VERY HIGH VELOCITY, THIN TARGET, LARGE, RAGGED EXIT.

F VELOCITY, CALIBER, AND THICKNESS OF TISSUE SUCH THAT CAVITATION OCCURS DEEP INSIDE AND ENTRANCE AND EXIT ARE SMALL.

G ASYMMETRIC CAVITATION AS BULLET BEGINS TO DEFORM AND TUMBLE.

H WOUND PREDICTED FOR ULTRA-HIGH-VELOCITY, SMALL-CALIBER PROJECTILES NOW UNDER DEVELOPMENT. NO EXIT WOUND. FRAGMENTATION OF BULLET.

Figure 2-1 A–H The variations of ballistic effects upon animal tissue are depicted schematically and separately defined.

of kinetic energy of the missile dissipated in the wound. A rifled bullet*
fired at low velocity, spinning with its long axis parallel to the trajectory
may pass rather cleanly through tissue and exit retaining most of the
kinetic energy it had upon impact. A high-velocity, rifled bullet of the
same caliber will likely strike with its long axis at an angle with respect
to its trajectory, and as a consequence of this and of its great velocity,
deform and even disintegrate in the tissue. The much greater tissue
resistance to this high-velocity, deformed, and "tilted" missile (Figure
2-1G) and its fragments leads to the degradation of an enormous
amount of kinetic energy. The tissue damage is proportionately great.

Kinetic energy of a missile is proportional to the mass of the missile
times the square of its velocity (KE $\sim$ MV^2). Tissue damage is proportional to the difference between the kinetic energy the missile has
upon impact and that on exit. The design of bullets has been directed
towards maximizing the difference between the kinetic energy of impact and exit, and thus increasing the damage these bullets inflict. The
Geneva Convention, prior to World War I, mandated that bullets be
copper-jacketed, i.e., that lead bullets be enclosed in copper, to
minimize their deformation on impact and minimize the resultant
tissue damage. Although this nicety has not seen its parallel in the
subsequent half-century of development of other military means of inflicting damage to human tissue, the Geneva Convention has been
strictly adhered to in succeeding wars. Non–copper-jacketed, *hollow-
point, soft-nose,* or *dum-dum* bullets and other technical means of promoting deformation of the bullet and increasing its profile perpen-
dicular to its trajectory following impact have been strictly avoided for
combat infantry around the world in the intervening 74 years. Curi-
ously, we have been less concerned in civilian life with limiting the
degradation in tissue of kinetic energy of bullets. Constraints such as
those specified in the Geneva Convention are not imposed upon ammunition used by private citizens or by law enforcement officers.
Copper-jacketed bullets are rarely fired from weapons in civilian
crime and, ironically, wounds inflicted by bullets fired in civilian life
today may be more severe and more threatening than those sustained
in military combat from bullets of comparable size and velocity.

Prior to World War II, the emphasis in the development of small
arms weapons and their ammunition was upon the mass of the missile.
An example is the U.S. military 45-caliber (11.4-mm), semiautomatic
pistol (Colt 45, M1911-A1 pistol), which was developed specifically
for "knock-down" capability in the Spanish-American War. This
weapon fires a relatively low velocity (860 ft/sec, or 262 m/sec) bullet
five times the weight of that fired by the M-16 rifle. Contrary to common belief, the lethality of this pistol is relatively modest. The M-16,

---

*A rifled bullet is an elongated projectile to which spin on its long axis has been imparted
by helical grooves in the barrel of the firearm.

firing a much smaller round at nearly four times the velocity of the round fired by the Colt 45, imparts nearly three times the kinetic energy. There is an additional feature which makes the M-16 rifle a far more lethal weapon than the Colt 45. When bullet velocities approach or exceed 3000 ft/sec, (914 m/sec), the bullets tend to become unstable in flight and may "yaw" or "tumble," as illustrated in Figures 2-2 and 2-3 respectively.

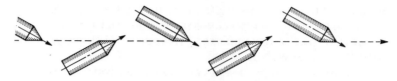

YAWING IS THE DEVIATION OF A BULLET IN ITS LONGITUDINAL AXIS FROM THE STRAIGHT LINE OF FLIGHT

Figure 2-2   The special ballistic property "yaw" associated with missiles of very high velocities (c 3000 feet per second) is depicted schematically.

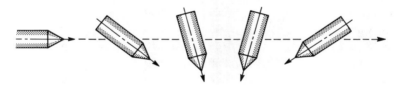

TUMBLING IS THE ACTION OF FORWARD ROTATION AROUND THE CENTER OF MASS

Figure 2-3   The special ballistic property "tumble" associated with missiles of very high velocities (c 3000 feet per second) is depicted schematically.

These phenomena increase the profile or projected transverse area of the missile as it strikes its target. Upon impact, and as a result of these factors, there is an inevitable increase in these motions, thus increasing the retarding force of the tissue and increasing the rate of dissipation of the kinetic energy of the bullet. A projectile moving in stable flight (Figure 2-1G), upon passing at high velocity from air into tissue a thousand times more dense, will tend to become unstable, to yaw, tumble, and fragment, dissipating its kinetic energy with great intensity. Thus, modern, high-velocity bullets tend to violate the intention of the Geneva Convention.

Tissue damage at any point along the track of the bullet, or of its fragments, is proportional to the rate of dissipation of kinetic energy

$(KE \sim M [V_{impact} - V_{exit}]^2)$, or the rate of its conversion into mechanical disruption of tissue. At low velocity, this rate is proportional to velocity squared. As velocity approaches and exceeds the speed of sound (1100 ft/sec or 335 m/sec), the rate of dissipation of kinetic energy becomes proportional to velocity cubed, or to even higher powers of velocity. Thus, tissue damage in a gunshot wound is much more sensitive to the velocity of the missile than to its mass. As designers of firearms and ammunition have sought higher velocities and smaller bullets, partly to produce flatter trajectories and achieve greater accuracy, and partly to facilitate the transport of ammunition and weapons, they have achieved the potential for exponentially increasing tissue destruction from weapons and ammunition of comparable size and weight.

The ballistic properties of common pistol rounds are summarized in Table 2-1, and those of three 22-caliber rifle rounds in Table 2-2.

Table 2-1
Ballistic Properties—Pistols*

Pistol	Bullet Weight (Grains)	Muzzle Velocity (ft/sec)	Kinetic Energy (ft-lbs)
25 Caliber	50	820	74
380 Caliber	95	955	190
38 Caliber	158	870	263
45 Caliber	250	860	406
38 Caliber (Super Vel)	110	1450	519

*The ballistic properties of bullets fired from common handguns (pistols or revolvers) are tabulated according to weapon (caliber), weight (grains), muzzle velocity (feet per second), and from these data, kinetic energy (foot/pounds) at the muzzle calculated.

Table 2-2
Ballistic Properties—22-Caliber Rifles*

Caliber	Model	Bullet Weight (Grains)	Muzzle Velocity (ft/sec)	Kinetic Energy (ft-lbs)
22	22 Long Rifle	40	1255	140
222	Hornet	50	3140	1094
223	M-16	55	3240	1282

*The ballistic properties of three 22†-caliber rifle bullets are tabulated according to caliber, weight (grains), muzzle velocity (feet per second), and from the latter two parameters, kinetic energy at the muzzle expressed in foot-pounds.
†22 includes any caliber between .220 and .230 inches.

With the exception of the "high-powered" handgun (38-caliber, Super Vel round), all of the handguns are, by definition, low-velocity, and the muzzle velocity translated into kinetic energy in each case is well below 1000 ft-lbs/sec. Conversely, all of the rifle rounds are traveling at muzzle velocities in excess of 1000 ft/sec; therefore, kinetic energy at the muzzle is considerably higher. In a comparison of the 22 long rifle with the M-16, an increase in muzzle velocity by a factor of 3 coincides with an increase in kinetic energy by a factor of almost 10. These data emphasize the importance of velocity, as compared to mass, in defining ballistic properties and predicting wounding capabilities of weapons.

CAVITATION

The second principle, cavitation as recognized by Woodruff in 1898,[1] concerns a momentary acceleration of tissue in a direction forward and laterally away from the track of the bullet. This acceleration generates a transient, water-vapor–filled cavity around the bullet and its track. The cavity may be many times the diameter of the bullet. Low-velocity missiles push the tissues aside and induce practically no cavitation (Figure 2-1A). When bullets of similar caliber, but of higher velocity, penetrate tissue, sufficient kinetic energy is transferred to the tissue to compress and accelerate it away from the surface of the bullet (Figure 2-1B) forming, within a few microseconds, a cavity around the bullet and its subsequent track. This cavity, which continues to enlarge after the bullet passes, is at subatmospheric pressure. Into it may be sucked foreign material and tissue fragments (secondary missiles). Within a few milliseconds, the cavity begins to collapse under atmospheric pressure, and tissues recoil. The cavity reforms and collapses a few more times at rapidly diminishing amplitude, until all imparted energy is dissipated. It is this alternating stretch and compression of tissue that adds substantially to the tissue damage in a wound from a high-velocity missile.

Cavitation develops readily and extensively in tissue with low tensile strength. Thus, cavitation develops more easily and extensively in parenchymal organs, such as the liver, than in striated muscle, and in the latter, more easily than in dense connective tissue, such as bone or tendon. In any microscopic region, because of the mix of fascia or stroma with more cellular tissue, anatomic distortions develop, and this further contributes to tissue disruption.

At even higher velocities, the initial cavity may be many centimeters in diameter and closer to the point of impact (Figure 2-1D). The volume of tissue damage will be greater. The entrance wound may be larger than the diameter of the bullet. If the target is relatively thin, the bullet may exit just as its yaw and deformation and consequent degradation of kinetic energy are beginning to impart sufficient energy to the tissue to induce cavitation. The result will be a large and ragged exit wound (Figure 2-1E). If the target is sufficiently thick, the maximal rate of degradation of kinetic energy may occur when the bullet is halfway through (Figure 2-1F). The cavity will be maximal deep within the target, and the entrance and exit wounds may appear as innocuous as those of a low-velocity wound. As the bullet tumbles and deforms, its kinetic energy is degraded even more rapidly. A larger and asymmetrical cavity will be generated (Figure 2-1G).

If the bullet fragments, there may be no exit wound. At the very high velocities of projectiles now under development, we can project that cavitation will be large and shallow, with explosive destruction extending many centimeters in all directions from the point of impact, and with no exit wound (Figure 2-1H).

Critical application of these two principles—the relation of mass and velocity of the projectile to its potential for imparting destructive forces to tissues and the mechanism of cavitation—will guide the surgeon in his or her appraisal of the extent of damage, the need for debridement, the potential for infection, as well as the possibilities for reconstruction. Obviously, management can be more effective if the surgeon can obtain appropriate information regarding the nature of the weapon inflicting the damage.

SUMMARY

With the exponential increase in muzzle velocity of firearms in this century, an understanding of wound ballistics is becoming of increasing importance in the management of gunshot wounds. Potential tissue damage is proportional to the square of the missile velocity, and high velocity drives tissue away from the missile track. This results in tensile, compressive, and shearing forces destroying tissue as far as several centimeters away from the actual track of the missile.

REFERENCES

1. Amato, J.J., Billy, L.J., Lawson, N.S. et al. High velocity missile injury. An experimental study of the retentive forces of tissue. *Am J Surg.* 127:454–459, 1974.

2. Charters, A.C., III, and Charters, A.C. Wounding mechanism of very high velocity projectiles. *J Trauma.* 16:464–470, 1976.

3. Berlin, R., Gelin, L.E., Janzon, B. et al. Local effects of assault rifle bullets in live tissues. *Acta Chir Scand.* 459(suppl):1–85, 1976.

4. Shuck, L.W., Orgel, M.G., and Vogel, A.V. Self inflicted .gunshot wounds to the face: A review of 15 cases. *J Trauma.* (In press) Presented at the 39th Annual Meeting of the American Association for the Surgery of Trauma. Chicago, September 13–15, 1979.

5. Rybeck, B., and Janzon, B. Absorption of missile energy in soft tissue. *Acta Chir Scand.* 142:201–207, 1976.

3 Emergency Management: Resuscitation

The patient was treated by teams of physicians. While one team operated to insert a tube into his leg for the administration of drugs and fluids, another team operated to clear the President's airway with a tracheostomy, which is an incision into the windpipe. Other teams of physicians monitored the patient's heart and lungs, his blood pressure and pulse, and his neurological status. In the next room, other teams of surgeons treated the Governor, who sustained a gunshot wound of the chest, requiring insertion of a chest tube known as a thoracostomy.*

The immediate treatment of a patient who has sustained a gunshot wound does not differ from that care rendered to any patient who is acutely ill and is received in the emergency treatment facility of a major medical installation. The concept "team approach" is never more appropriate than in this phase of the patient's evaluation and care. The ideal team consists of several surgeons, an anesthesiologist or

*Report of the Commission on the Assassination of President John F. Kennedy, 1966.

anesthetist, several nurses, and several nursing assistants. Together, these individuals initiate a rapid evaluation of the patient's respiratory, cardiovascular, and nervous systems.

It is appropriate, depending upon the number of casualties received, for a triage officer to be appointed, presumably prior to the reception of the patients.* Depending upon the size of the treatment facility, more than one severely injured individual can constitute a triage situation. The triage officer's responsibility is only in the orderly flow of patient care and the identification of shortages of those resources necessary for adequate patient resuscitation, treatment, and, in certain circumstances, evacuation. He does not involve himself in direct patient management. The triage officer is usually a senior surgeon, but the role also may be adequately filled by a senior resident in surgery. By definition, the triage officer is in overall charge of patient care, and all else within the treatment facility is subject to the results of his decisions. He identifies the injury, assigns the surgical team to the patient's resuscitation, and determines the orders of priority with regard to radiographic evaluation and operating room scheduling. In addition, he calls upon the hospital's medical director and administrative chief for support of additional medical personnel and/or paramedical resources such as blood bank and radiologic techniques and equipment. The triage officer is the key to successful management of multiple casualties.

With a well-staffed, experienced, and well-rehearsed team, it is usually possible to attend to a spectrum of major problems in each patient more or less concurrently. With a smaller and less experienced team, priorities in resuscitation must be established. Respiration and circulation are usually of first priority and are best addressed simultaneously.

Impairment of respiration due to obstruction of the airway must be distinguished from that due to derangements of the ventilatory mechanism secondary to such conditions as flail chest, hemopneumothorax, or paralysis of the respiratory muscles. Where the patient's ability to ventilate adequately is questionable, the insertion of an

---

*Triage (from the French, *trier*—to sort)—the sorting of patients for priority care when numbers overburden ordinary medical resources and personnel. Usually three categories are established: 1) Patients whose wounds are not life-threatening and who can survive without hospitalization are often referred to as "the walking wounded." In a mass casualty, they would be told to return for care in 24 to 48 hours, conditions permitting. 2) "The expectant" are those patients who are probably fatally injured. Their injuries are such that even heroic measures will not likely result in meaningful survival. They are treated with a minimum of resources, made as comfortable as possible, and their early demise is anticipated. 3) Patients who can probably be saved if immediate, definitive care is rendered, and if resources and personnel concentrate on their care, are often called "the priority."

Napoleon's surgeon, Larrey, is given credit for the popularization of the concept of triage.

endotracheal tube is indicated. In the event that the gunshot wound involves the neck or maxillofacial area, it may be necessary to perform an immediate tracheostomy to clear the airway. If, on the other hand, the patient's respiratory rate and the color of skin and mucous membranes appear adequate, as is often the case, then no ventilatory assistance is required. The importance of periodic reassessment of the patient's respiratory function cannot be overemphasized.

Control of external hemorrhage is an obvious priority. It is usually accomplished before the patient reaches the trauma team and for obvious reasons. Digital pressure upon actively bleeding exposed parts is the surest preliminary measure preceding more adequate control with appropriate surgical instruments. In the case of severe hemorrhage from an extremity such as that associated with traumatic amputation, a pneumatic tourniquet is indicated and should be available in the emergency room. The tourniquet should be appropriately placed proximally on the extremity and inflated to 300 mm Hg for the upper extremity, and 600 mm Hg for the lower extremity. The pneumatic tourniquet should stay in place until it is possible to control the hemorrhage adequately with more definitive measures. The pneumatic tourniquet deserves a place with portable emergency equipment organized for the treatment of trauma, space permitting.

An additional technique which has been employed successfully in management of exsanguinating hemorrhage in the field is the MAST (Medical Anti-Shock Trousers) unit. This device has been successfully applied at the roadside to patients sustaining multiple injuries to the lower extremities, pelvis, and abdomen. It also can be successfully utilized during early resuscitation in a variety of medical emergencies.

For similar reasons, appropriate techniques for splinting long-bone fractures are indicated within the resuscitation area. The pneumatic splint is a well-accepted technique for immobilizing fractures of both lower and upper extremities. The adage, "splint them where they lie," still applies to the in-hospital situation in which the fracture of a long bone is identified, perhaps for the first time following the patient's injury.

Hemorrhage from the maxillofacial region is best managed with immediate surgical exploration, under general anesthesia. Hemorrhage from a scalp laceration can best be taken care of with suture closure of the laceration without undue attention to sterile technique or local anesthesia. Evidence of significant and excessive hemorrhage from within the thoracic, abdominal, or pelvic cavities, of course requires more extensive evaluation. If surgical intervention appears necessary, it is best managed in optimal surgical circumstances, namely, the surgical operating suite.

In patients who have sustained acute penetrating trauma to the trunk or extremities, the pulse and systemic arterial pressure are the best initial indicators of the adequacy of cardiovascular function.

Here, the team leader must make certain that the individual monitoring the patient's arterial pressure is capable, reliable, and conscientious, since vital signs can deteriorate within minutes of a recently recorded normal determination. If any doubt exists as to the competence of the paramedical personnel, then a physician should be assigned to the specific task of monitoring vital signs. The frequency of observation and documentation of vital signs cannot be overemphasized. In the acutely ill, they are often measured as frequently as several times per minute.

Simultaneously, a rapid, yet thorough neurologic examination is indicated, particularly when the gunshot wound appears to have involved the trunk, neck, or head. This part of the examination can be accomplished literally within seconds, and includes an evaluation of vital signs, pupils, motor and sensory function in upper and lower extremities, and deep tendon reflexes. Characteristically, a space-occupying lesion resulting from intracranial accumulation of a relatively small amount of blood produces systemic arterial hypertension, a widening of the pulse pressure, and bradycardia. Presumably, bradycardia is secondary to hypertension. Although its exact cause is unknown, hypertension usually reflects brain-stem herniation and interference with cardioregulatory centers in the medulla. An alternate explanation is related to the increased intracranial pressure producing a reflex increase in intravascular pressure to compensate for the inadequate perfusion of the brain. In an otherwise healthy young male with a normal systemic arterial pressure of 110/70 mm Hg, the appearance of a systolic pressure of 180 mm Hg and a diastolic pressure of 90 mm Hg characterizes an acute increase in intracranial pressure. When these observations are accompanied by evidence of bradycardia in the neighborhood of 48 to 66, suspicions should be aroused. If these findings are present, then in all likelihood, the respiratory rate may be well below normal and suggest that the patient's neurologic status is being dramatically compromised. Simultaneously, abnormalities in thermal regulation may be manifested by an abnormally high or low core temperature. Time usually does not permit the documentation of this parameter, and measurement of temperature is usually not decisive in the patient's initial management.

Usually there is a fixed dilated pupil on the side of the source of increased intracranial pressure. This sign indicates paralysis of the pupillary constrictor muscle due to compression of parasympathetic preganglionic axons in the oculomotor (Cranial III) nerve. In such displacement of the brain, this nerve is usually compressed between the uncus of the temporal lobe and the free border of the tentorium cerebelli, as may also be the abducens (Cranial VI) nerve. In this process, the development of a fixed dilated pupil may soon be followed by inability to abduct (laterally deviate) the eye. With greater compression of the oculomotor nerve, more general oculomotor paralysis develops ipsilaterally. In all likelihood, these observations will be associated with contralateral hemiparesis and a contralateral hemisensory defect. On this same side, there may be hyperreflexia and abnormal reflexes such as those described by Babinski. These long-track signs reflect pressure upon the cerebral peduncle by the free edge of the tentorium. These assessments can be made rapidly, usually by questioning the patient as to his ability to move upper and lower extremities and having him describe sensation in response to painful stimuli. If the patient's condition has deteriorated to the point that he is unable to respond to questions, then gross approximation of these parameters will be necessary. Absence of these neurologic signs and symptoms is as important for documentation purposes as is their presence, since not only can neurologic signs change abruptly within the emergency room, but also the absence of a neurologic defect may be important in evaluating the possibility of a cervical spinal-cord injury, should there exist the probability of a cervical spine fracture or dislocation. A high index of suspicion of surgical spinal injury is necessary when evaluating any patient with significant trauma, as well as patients with apparently minor scalp lacerations.

Assuming that the brief neurologic examination is negative, and assuming the patient exhibits no signs or symptoms suggestive of a spinal fracture such as tenderness or pain over the spinal column, then it is appropriate to proceed with a more thorough examination. In the management of an obvious gunshot wound, all of the patient's clothes must be removed and the entire body examined for the presence of additional entrance or exit wounds. Entrance and exit wounds are most commonly overlooked in hairy regions such as the scalp and the perineum. Exit wounds provide insight into the probable path of the missile and suggest appropriate diagnostic studies. A good rule of thumb is that "one body cavity above and one below" any entrance or exit wound should be viewed radiographically from anteroposterior (A-P) and lateral positions to determine the presence or absence of metallic foreign bodies within a body cavity. A metallic foreign body within the neck or abdomen, by itself, is an indication for mandatory exploration of the neck or abdomen. Fragments within the pelvis call for exploratory laparotomy. Following a gunshot wound, a metallic foreign body within the cranial cavity is an indication for craniectomy and debridement, depending upon the neurologic status of the patient. The same is not necessarily true for metallic foreign bodies within the chest, as will be discussed.

While the above is being accomplished, members of the surgical team insert appropriate tubes for therapy, physiologic monitoring, and diagnosis. These tubes include large-bore, intravenous catheters for administration of electrolyte solutions, drugs, blood, and blood components, as well as for monitoring central venous pressure. Measurement of cardiac output by thermodilution utilizing a Swan-Ganz catheter in the pulmonary artery presently is not practicable within most emergency rooms, even those in trauma centers. In the near future, however, the patient's initial resuscitation may well include the implementation of such sophisticated techniques of physiologic monitoring. Whether the intravenous catheters are placed in the saphenous vein at the level of the groin, or at the ankle, is of small concern, bearing in mind that injuries to major veins in the trunk contraindicate the resuscitation with fluid replacement through these lines. An alternative is a subclavian venous catheter, or jugular venous catheter, or, in fact, a catheter placed by way of a brachial vein in the antecubital fossa. The best approach is to use more than one access route and to include at least one access route in the upper extremities and one in the lower extremities. A radial arterial catheter is not usually used in the emergency room, but on the other hand, it is a sophisticated approach to the careful, continuous monitoring of systemic arterial pressure.

A Foley catheter is almost always indicated in the management of a gunshot wound. The size of catheter or its balloon is not important, but the catheter serves two important functions: (1) diagnosis of penetrating genitourinary tract injury, and (2) management of renal function during shock. It is unusual to have a penetrating injury to the genitourinary tract without the appearance of blood, usually bright red, in the drainage from the Foley catheter inserted transurethrally into the bladder. Why the blood is usually bright red is beyond the concern of this discussion. When it occurs, hematuria is usually gross. Grossly clear urine exiting the catheter is an indication of probable integrity of the genitourinary tract. It is likely that a patient sustaining a gunshot wound of the trunk or proximal extremities will require major surgery and moderately long hospitalization, during which time the adequacy of renal function can be measured by urinary output.

Also, a gunshot wound of the trunk is an indication for insertion of a nasogastric (Levin) tube. This maneuver is important for several reasons: (1) the patient invariably has a fairly full stomach, which warrants at least some attempt at decompression, realizing that it is difficult to remove solid food through any size of nasogastric tube known; and (2) although it is much less common to diagnose penetrating injuries to the gastrointestinal tract on the basis of drainage from the Levin tube, the appearance of blood in the Levin tube nonetheless raises the suspicion of this particular injury and is an indication by itself for exploratory laparotomy. A perhaps more subtle use of the Levin tube is its radiographic appearance following insertion in the assessment of possible diaphragmatic injury and herniation of intra-abdominal contents into the chest. Almost invariably, this is related to an injury to the left hemidiaphragm and displacement of the stomach into the left pleural space. This complication of both thoracic and abdominal gunshot wounds, which is difficult to diagnose, may prove fatal if overlooked. Likewise, injuries to the thoracic esophagus may become apparent only when the nasogastric tube is seen to be present in either the right or left pleural cavity rather than in the stomach, despite passage of a significant length of the tube. The corollary, absence of sanguineous drainage from a nasogastric tube does not, by any means, rule out the possibility of injury to the stomach or neighboring parts of the gastrointestinal tract. All too frequently, in fact, a significant injury to the stomach, including through-and-through penetration is unaccompanied by sanguineous, nasogastric Levin tube drainage. Doubt as to the existence of a penetrating injury to the gastrointestinal tract can be illuminated by the injection of water-soluble contrast material through the Levin tube and radiographic observation for extravasation. This technique is probably most applicable to the possible injuries of the thoracic esophagus rather than to the gastrointestinal tract located in the abdomen.

While it is generally considered mandatory that penetrating gunshot wounds of the head, neck, and abdomen be explored surgically, the same is not true of penetrating injuries of the chest. Evaluation of a thoracic gunshot wound is based upon the clinical determination of diminution in breath sounds on the suspected side. This finding is an indication for insertion of a chest tube or a tube thoracostomy.

If the patient's vital signs are normal and stable and a question remains regarding the possible presence of significant intrathoracic injury, radiographic evaluation of the chest is indicated. If the radiogram is sought prior to tube thoracostomy, then a physician must accompany the patient during the procedure in order to detect the development of complications of chest penetration. When in doubt, tube thoracostomy, not thoracentesis, is indicated. The vast majority (85%) of penetrating thoracic injuries respond to tube thoracostomy alone. The surgical team in the emergency room should be alert to the possible need for immediate thoracostomy when there is continuing blood loss through the chest tube, when the color of the chest tube drainage is bright red, when the patient sustains cardiac arrest, or when injury to the heart or great vessels is suspected.

When the patient's condition permits, the need for exploring the abdomen can be more precisely determined using the following procedures: (1) probing the wound; (2) exploring the wound under local anesthesia; (3) "stabagram"; (4) peritoneal lavage; (5) demonstrating signs of peritoneal inflammation, which may be secondary to intra-abdominal hemorrhage. These will be discussed in more detail in Chapter 7.

The size of the resuscitation area and its facilities will reflect the casualty admission rate. Most large urban hospitals that provide care for trauma victims in the United States today find that a centrally located room with two to four stretchers is appropriate for most situations. This trauma room contains units for intubation and assisted ventilation, cardiac rate and rhythm monitors, cardiac defibrillation devices, "cut-down" trays, tracheostomy sets, tube thoracostomy trays, and intravenous fluids for immediate administration.

Although there is a controversy regarding the appropriate fluid for resuscitation when acute intravascular blood-volume reduction is probably secondary to blood loss, it is reasonable to plan resuscitation with crystalloid or plasma, and ultimately, whole blood. Studies during the Vietnam War indicated that between two and three units of whole blood were required per hospitalized patient and that for those transfused, the figure ranged from four to nine units, with a mean of approximately seven.[1]

Whereas in previous wars, blood for transfusion was mostly type O, in the Vietnam War, transfusion eventually became almost always with type-specific whole blood. In Vietnam, crystalloid, or colloid blood substitutes, were used to the extent of two and one-half times that of whole blood.[1]

Ideally, type-specific, low titer, refrigerated whole blood should be available in the resuscitation area. Today, it is possible to determine the patient's blood type and transfuse him with type-specific whole blood within 30 seconds of his arrival. Although this capability is little appreciated, nor widely exploited in the United States today, it was routinely accomplished in Vietnam over a decade ago. Three forms of blood replacement are possible: (1) type O negative (universal donor) blood; (2) type-specific, uncrossmatched blood; (3) crossmatched blood. It is unusual in most treatment facilities, even where trauma is treated on a daily basis, for crossmatched blood to be available in less than 30 to 45 minutes. If type-specific whole blood is not immediately available and transfusion is indicated immediately, use of type O blood must be accepted. However, if more than five units of type O blood have been administered to a patient whose blood type is ultimately determined to be other than O, then type O blood replacement should be continued. The reason is the danger of intravascular cross reaction between the two types of transfused blood if a second blood type is subsequently administered. The resuscitation team must remain cognizant of these logistical problems during the early decisions in patient management, when hemorrhagic hypotension is present. In the future, substitutes such as hemoglobin solution may obviate the need for identification of the patient's blood type, let alone the necessity for crossmatching. At present, these blood substitutes are sufficiently experimental to preclude their usage in the management of resuscitation following gunshot wounds.

The resuscitation team must be prepared to apply appropriate antibiotics at the earliest indication. Some believe antibiotics should be administered prophylactically on admission to reduce the incidence of infection.[2] After serious injury we recommend broad-spectrum antibiotic therapy parenterally and in high dose soon after admission even though the evidence for such is presently lacking.

Tetanus immunization should be administered during the resuscitation of a patient who has sustained a gunshot wound. Although almost all United States citizens have been given adequate immunization to tetanus, the disease still occurs in this country and remains prevalent abroad.[3] The fatality rate remains about 50%. The concept of the "tetanus prone," or "dirty," wound persists and holds that certain wounds are more susceptible to infection by *Clostridium tetani* and, therefore, should be treated differently regarding tetanus prophylaxis.[3] Recent experience in the management of large numbers of Vietnamese civilians who did not receive tetanus immunization as part of a program, or associated with a previous injury, indicated that a rate of tetanus of approximately 80% followed "minor" or "clean" wounds. (K. Arnold, personal communication, March 1975). In any event, the gunshot wound is by definition a "dirty" wound. Tetanus toxoid should be administered and the small possibility of allergic reactions to tetanus toxoid accepted. Current tetanus prophylaxis assumes previous immunization and includes administration of a booster dose of 0.5 ml of tetanus toxoid intramuscularly as soon as resuscitative efforts permit. Often the patient is unable to give an adequate or accurate immunization history. Prior U.S. military service is a reliable indication of previous immunization to tetanus, and adequate antibody titers can be demonstrated as a result of a single booster shot ten years or more following the most recent immunization. If prior immunization has not been instituted, or if history is doubtful, then 500 units of human immune globulin should be given intramuscularly along with active immunization.[4]

When the missile appears to have inflicted injury to more than one organ or system, involving more than one surgical subspecialty, it is customary, and probably wise, that a general surgeon be in overall charge. With increasing specialization, injuries involving specific surgical subspecialties tend to be dealt with to the exclusion of consideration for possible injuries elsewhere. This must be avoided.

The equipment in a modern treatment facility necessary to perform the emergency resuscitation of a patient sustaining a gunshot wound includes a readily available room for resuscitation which, in all aspects, simulates an operating room. It contains equipment appropriate for immediate tracheostomy, thoracostomy, peritoneal lavage, along with tubes for insertion into appropriate body cavities and blood vessels. In addition, adequate lighting, wall suction, and oxygen, as well as the instrumentation and assistance to perform a laparotomy or thoracotomy are required.

Important medicolegal aspects pertain to the treatment of many gunshot wounds, whether incurred in peacetime or combat. Law enforcement officials are constantly frustrated by the apparent careless manner in which critical information or evidence is handled even by experienced medical and paramedical personnel in the emergency room, as well as in the operating room. While a formal "standard operating procedure"[5] that would satisfy the criminologist concerned with the medical aspects of a gunshot wound has been proposed, such SOP would probably confound even the most cooperative and concerned trauma center team. Nonetheless, certain principles deserve reiteration and emphasis, since the present legal climate of this country places very stringent constraints upon the law enforcement community.

"Each instance of a frustration of justice due to careless handling of evidence by a surgical team is an irony not to be tolerated."[6] At the bare minimum, the medical team receiving a patient who has sustained a gunshot wound should: (1) exert care not to destroy clothing worn by the patient, and, in particular, cut around and not through bullet holes in clothing; (2) carefully preserve and turn over to appropriate law enforcement officials any weapon, and more specifically, any metallic foreign body, such as a bullet or its fragments; (3) describe as precisely as possible and even photograph prior to debridement (a diagram for the patient's permanent record is an appropriate alternative) any entrance or exit wound; and (4) query the patient and witnesses as to the nature of the weapon (firearm, caliber, missile, load), direction, distance, number of assailants, number of rounds fired and received, etc. Although the surgical team is not expected to assume the role of sleuth, its cooperation may well prove critical to the pursuit of justice.

Equally important, an accurate appraisal of the mechanism of injury is an integral part of the history and physical examination which necessarily precedes the meaningful medical management of any illness, regardless of its etiology. For example, the entrance wound inflicted by a small zip gun (22-caliber pistol) will be indistinguishable from that caused by the most advanced of standard military rifles (M-16), and yet the damage caused by these two weapons will be remarkably dissimilar. Likewise, if "the usual 38-caliber pistol wound" was, in fact, caused by a 38-caliber, Super Vel round, the damage inflicted will be similarly disparate, and the anticipation of this damage will be to the advantage of both physician and patient.

SUMMARY

In summary, the determination of survival of a victim of a gunshot wound is often made during his resuscitation, whether in the field or in the emergency room of a major trauma center. A well-trained, well-rehearsed team approach to such patients is critical. Also essential to survival, depending upon the number of injured, is the concept of triage. Prior identification of the triage officer should eliminate potential problems relating to logistics of casualty management. Priorities in resuscitation include ascertaining an adequate airway, maintenance of adequate cardiovascular function, identification of potential for neurologic damage, and control of hemorrhage. All of these priorities must be addressed virtually simultaneously if success is to be anticipated. Only a team approach can provide this anticipation. The team includes surgeons, nurses, an anesthesiologist (or anesthetist), and other paramedical personnel. A radiologist and a clinical pathologist ideally complement the team. Administrative personnel are also essential team members, but all are temporarily under direction of the triage officer if casualty load is impressive.

Immediate concern regards the airway, which is established by whatever means necessary. These range from nothing in the case of apparent normal respiration in a victim of trauma, to tracheostomy when a severe maxillofacial wound results from gunshot. Lesser procedures have been defined. Hemorrhage from an extremity may require a pneumatic tourniquet in the field or in the emergency room. Digital pressure can usually control bleeding from all sources of hemorrhage outside the trunk. Intravenous lines are mandatory and should be of large bore and inserted into both upper and lower extremities. A nasogastric (Levin) tube and transurethral bladder (Foley) catheter are almost always indicated for diagnostic and therapeutic reasons.

A rapid, precise neurologic examination must precede patient movement assuming other major concerns have been obviated. Careful examination of the patient includes removal of all clothing and examination for additional entrance and exit wounds. Areas where these are missed most frequently include the hair-bearing parts (i.e., scalp, axillae, and perineum). Rectal exam is mandatory since blood on the examining finger by itself mandates colostomy. Radiograms must be obtained in the anterior-posterior and lateral positions of each body cavity above and below an entrance or exit wound, assuming patient tolerance. Resuscitation with blood volume replacement may initially be Ringer's lactate solution, but should proceed immediately to whole blood when significant loss of such is inferred.[7] Type-specific blood and principles of its use should be available in the emergency room. Prophylaxis against tetanus and use of antibiotics should begin in the emergency room. Patient reassurance and relative consultation also belong in this phase of patient care when possible.

If more than one surgical or medical specialty is involved in the management of the victim of a gunshot wound, then overall management and thus responsibility belongs to the general or trauma surgeon. He orchestrates patient evaluation and management in concert with the triage officer when the patient load so indicates.

28

REFERENCES

1. Mendelson, J.A. The use of whole blood and blood volume expanders in U.S. military medical facilities in Vietnam, 1966-1971. *J Trauma.* 15:1-13, 1975.

2. Altemeier, W.A. The significance of infection in trauma. *Bull Am Coll Surg.* 57:7-16, 1972.

3. Rothstein, R.J., and Baker, F.J. Medical emergency management. Tetanus: prevention and treatment. *JAMA.* 240:675-676, 1978.

4. Faust R.A., Vickers, O.R., and Cohn, I. Tetanus: 2449 cases in 68 years at Charity Hospital. *J Trauma.* 16:704-712, 1976.

5. Godley, D.R., and Smith, T.K. Some medicolegal aspects of gunshot wounds. *J Trauma.* 17:866-871, 1977.

6. Harris, L.S. Editorial Comment. *J Trauma.* 17:871, 1977.

7. Sheldon, G.F., Watkins, G.M., Glover, J.L. et al. Present use of blood and blood products. *J Trauma.* (In press). Presented at the 39th Annual Meeting of the American Association for the Surgery of Trauma. Chicago, September 13-15, 1979.

4 The Head

A direct gunshot wound to the brain was generally fatal. If a soldier receiving such a wound was still alive upon admission to the hospital, he was usually in a terminal state. Only those who had been struck by a spent round or had received glancing or through-and-through frontal lobe bullet wounds remained neurologically viable enough to warrant surgical debridement.*

Two United States Presidents were assassinated by gunshot wounds of the head. On April 14, 1865, Abraham Lincoln was killed by what would now be classified as a low-velocity handgun. The weapon used was a derringer pistol, which fired a 44-caliber, "hand made ball of stout metal through a rifled barrel in a percussion cap ignition system with approximately 10 grains of black powder."[1] In contrast, the weapon that killed John F. Kennedy, on November 22, 1963,

---

*Carey, M.E., Young, H.F., and Mathis, J.L. The neurosurgical treatment of craniocerebral missile wounds in Vietnam. *Surg Gynecol Obstet.* 135:386–390, 1972.

almost 100 years later, was a relatively high-velocity rifle (Mannlicher-Carcano), which fired a 6.5-mm (25-caliber), 160-grain bullet with a muzzle velocity of approximately 2500 ft/sec (762 m/sec).[2]

The round that hit Lincoln was fired from a distance of approximately 2 ft; that from which Kennedy died, a distance of approximately 250 ft. Lincoln sustained a gunshot wound to his left occipital region, whereas President Kennedy sustained his wound to the right occipital region. In each case the degree of cranial damage led to a fatal prognosis by those in immediate attendance. Nearly a century of surgical research and experience had apparently not improved the prognosis for extensive brain injury, despite heroic measures at resuscitation.

Although the weapons utilized in these two assassinations represent two ends of a spectrum of ballistic performance, they nevertheless resulted in death. The apparent similarity of the two wounds is, however, misleading. Lincoln's wound was characterized by a single entrance and no exit; only one fragment of the bullet fired from the gun of John Wilkes Booth separated from the main round, which was otherwise found intact at autopsy within the President's cranial cavity. Conversely, the much smaller, .6.5-mm, round fired by Lee Harvey Oswald, while producing a similarly small entrance wound, caused in addition a massive exit wound, as was apparent in the Zapruder film and to those accompanying the President. The motorcycle escort, following the President's limousine, was doused with the resultant cloud of brain tissue exploding from the exit wound in the right parietal region. This wound was almost instantly fatal, although resuscitative efforts persisted for the subsequent 30 minutes. Lincoln, in contrast, survived for nine hours beyond the time of injury.

The first bullet fired by Oswald, which struck Kennedy approximately five seconds prior to the fatal wound, penetrated his neck from posterior to anterior and injured his cervical spine, trachea, esophagus, and right apical pleura. This undoubtedly would not have been a fatal wound, as some have speculated, despite the apparent injury to the sixth cervical vertebral body and possibly to the cervical spinal cord. The force of this missile is evident from the fact that it went on to penetrate then-Governor John Connally's right chest, causing a through-and-through wound which required thoracotomy and pulmonary lobectomy. The round then penetrated the Governor's right wrist causing a comminuted fracture of the right radius, expending itself essentially intact in his right thigh. The missile which inflicted all this damage had a muzzle velocity 2300 to 2500 ft/sec and would be classed as of intermediate to high velocity. This is well below that now employed by the United States Army with its M-16 rifle (muzzle velocity 3240 ft/sec, or 988 m/sec) and commercially available rifles used for hunting big game (where muzzle velocities can easily approach 5000 ft/sec) (1524 m/sec).

As discussed in Chapter 2, doubling the muzzle velocity quadruples the energy of the missile. It is probable that the much smaller bullet that struck Kennedy and Connally weighed less than half that fired by Booth at Lincoln yet had a muzzle velocity three times greater. The smaller bullet thus imparted on impact a kinetic energy five times greater. The devastating blow which literally exploded Kennedy's right cerebral hemisphere resulted in a counterforce that drove the President's head to his rear and left, in such a fashion as to draw much speculation as to whether an additional assassin had fired a round forward of the President.

HISTORY OF MANAGEMENT

Management of high velocity missile wounds of the head usually demands a high degree of special expertise. The following discussion is in no way intended to develop some of that expertise, but is intended to review for the generalist the state of the art, the degree and types of salvage that are possible, and some of the directions in which he can go for help.

As in the case of fatal gunshot wounds of the chest, those of the head accounted for a disproportionately high fraction of the total fatal gunshot wounds suffered in the Vietnam and Korean Wars. The respective figures were 39% and 41%,[3] although the fractional silhouette is only about 10% when considered in terms of the frontal silhouette of the body.

As indicated in Table 4-1, the mortality from intracranial wounds* approached 75% prior to World War I. Cushing[4] documented in World War I a progressive decline in the mortality rate associated with wounds involving dural penetration. His personal series of 133 cases, treated during a three-month period in 1917, had a mortality of 55% for the first third of the cases, 41% for the second third, and 29% for the final third. From this brief but intensive experience, Cushing advocated debridement of bone, brain, and metal followed by primary wound (but not dural) closure. He emphasized the importance of early operation although due to delays in transport few of the patients in his series underwent definitive surgery until 12 hours after injury. Many were not operated upon until more than 24 hours after wounding. Including late deaths, Cushing's overall operative mortality was 36%. This remarkable figure antedated the use of antibiotics, blood transfusions, and the concept of dural closure.

---

*What has often been called "craniocerebral wound" we will refer to as intracranial wound (including brain and other structures within the cranial cavity), since the former term has been used ambiguously.

Table 4-1
Mortality From Craniocerebral Wounds Incurred During
Military Combat

Conflict	No. Patients Analyzed	Mortality (%)	Reference
Crimean War*	878	74	G. McLeod, *Notes on the Surgery of the War in the Crimea, with Remarks on the Treatment of Gunshot Wounds.* Phildelphia: J.B. Lippincott, Co., 1862.
Civil War*	704	72	Med-Surg History of War of Rebellion, USGPO (1870–1878).
World War I	–	41	(4)
World War II	500	11	(7)
Korean War	673	10	J. Coates, and A. Meirowsky, *Neurological Surgery of Trauma.* (Washington, D.C.: USGPO, 1965) pp. 103–130.
Vietnam War	1732	9	(13)

*Nonoperative mortality.

Cushing's success in the management of intracranial trauma, later to be matched with his ultimate success in the management of intracranial tumors, was a neurosurgical milestone. From as early as 900 B.C., penetrating head injuries carried a 75% mortality, a rate that did not change significantly through the ages and subsequent conflicts including the Crimean War and the American Civil War.[5]

The experience of neurosurgeons in World War II led to a further significant reduction in mortality and to the introduction of additional principles of management of intracranial wounds. Small and Turner[6] reported a mortality of 16% in 500 patients operated upon between 1944 and 1945, during which time primary dural closure was neither advocated nor practiced. It was recognized that there could be relatively greater damage near the wound of exit than near the wound of entrance. A separate and additional craniectomy and debridement were advocated when a metallic fragment could be demonstrated to have crossed the midline and come to rest near the inner table overlying the brain opposite the wound of entrance.[7]

In the Korean War (1950–1953), with faster evacuation, more sophisticated antibiotic therapy, and greater availability of whole blood, primary closure of the dura at the time of initial debridement was evaluated, and found to reduce the incidence of infection and to facilitate definitive cranioplasty. However, it did not reduce the incidence of posttraumatic epilepsy.[8]

The incidence of intracranial hematoma in penetrating head wounds rose from about 4%[9] in World War II to about 46%[10] in the Korean War. The major reason for this difference was the faster evacuation and the greater probability of reaching definitive neurosurgical care in the Korean War. Also, during this conflict it became evident that the incidence of hematoma complicating intracranial trauma was significantly lower when the wounded were evacuated to Japan, as early in the war, rather than to neurosurgical teams within Korea, as later in the war. The converse was true of the incidence [11,12] of meningocerebral infection complicating intracranial wounds. Analysis of these data indicate that the longer time required for evacuation to Japan resulted in fewer survivors of more serious intracranial wounds. In general, this Korean experience documented an inverse relation between time from wounding to definitive neurosurgical care and incidence of intracranial hematoma, and a direct relation between this time and the incidence of meningocerebral infection following intracranial wounds. Presumably, the relatively longer time for evacuation permitted a hematoma to progress to a fatal extent and to favor the development of infection. The combination of evacuation by helicopter air ambulance and the forward deployment of definitive neurosurgical capability, although relatively primitive by today's standards, were two large steps forward in the military management of intracranial head wounds.

In the Vietnam War there was little apparent further reduction in mortality associated with intracranial head wounds. Among 2187 such patients treated at an evacuation hospital and reviewed by Hammon,[13] 455, or 21%, died shortly after reception and were not operated upon. Of the remaining 1732, all of whom were operated upon, 11.2% died. One-third of the patients in this series were civilians in whom the mortality was higher. This relatively unchanged mortality between the Korean and Vietnam wars reflects the greater air evacuation capability in Vietnam. Ninety-five percent of the patients reported by Hammon were brought to the 24th Evac Hospital in Long Binh by helicopter. Thus, the relatively more seriously ill "made it" to the hospital, and the neurosurgeons there were faced with a higher percentage of patients, some of whom in earlier wars probably would not have received definitive neurosurgical treatment. Rapid air evacuation in Vietnam provided for better care, but reduced the apparent success rate of the care. One report from Vietnam concluded that if the time interval between moment of injury and neurosurgical care exceeded 90 minutes, ". . . clinical deterioration occurred."[14]

The neurosurgeon in Vietnam learned what probably will remain for some time the current philosophy of care for penetrating brain injuries resulting from missiles. These principles include: (1) rapid resuscitation, (2) adequate debridement of all accessible injured tissues, (3) removal of all intracerebral bone fragments, (4) removal of all accessible metallic fragments and all intraventricular or intracisternal fragments, (5) primary closure of the dura and scalp, (6) careful postoperative radiography to rule out retained bone fragments, (7) prompt reoperation to remove retained bone fragments, and (8) prophylactic antibiotics and anticonvulsants.[14,15]

If these lessons from recent U.S. military experience are to be applied in the management of penetrating head injuries of peacetime, at least one very important principle must be kept in mind. The ratio of fragment wounds to bullet wounds was well above unity in the wars and the reported series referred to above. In civilian practice in the United States, the reverse is the case, since those sources of "fragment wounds" (mines, bombs, rockets, artillery, grenades) are far less commonly encountered than are gunshot wounds. As Carey has emphasized, ". . . a gunshot wound of the brain is generally fatal,"[15] and civilian experience has borne this out. In a recent report by Raimondi and Samuelson,[16] 30% of patients admitted alive to a large city hospital with a diagnosis of craniocerebral gunshot wound died of their injury. The operative mortality in this series was 15.5%. An even more recent report places this operative mortality even higher (22%), and advises against neurosurgical intervention for cases in which the patient is comatose and nonresponsive on admission.[17] All of such patients in the Hubschmann series succumbed whether they had surgery or not. In experimental craniocerebral missile injuries in primates, systemic arterial pressure correlates less well with prognosis than does carotid arterial blood flow.[18]

Today, high-velocity gunshot wounds of the head and face can be treated by debridement and primary closure, rather than by debridement and delayed primary closure as in most other regions of the body. As soon as possible, radiograms of the skull should be obtained. Internal ricochet of penetrating gunshot wounds of the skull has been documented, and the clinician should be cognizant of this phenomenon. It may explain discrepancies between the presumed path of a bullet and the clinical findings.[19] Often special views are needed to demonstrate injuries to the mandible, maxillofacial regions, and the base of the skull. Usually primary closure is not only well tolerated, presumably because of the generous blood supply to the head, but also necessary for maximizing cosmetic reconstitution.

MANAGEMENT

The Brain

In general, the presence of intracranial metallic fragments (Figures 4-1–4-3) and depressed skull fractures remains an indication for neurosurgical craniectomy, brain debridement, and primary closure of the dura to achieve a watertight (cerebrospinal fluid) seal reinforced by primary closure of the overlying fascia, muscle, and skin.[20] Elevation of a depressed skull fracture is essential to prevent a brain abscess, although studies from the Vietnam War revealed that many of the in-driven bone fragments were, in fact, sterile.* Whether their removal minimizes scar formation and epilepsy is moot since the neurosurgical procedure in itself can be a cause for posttraumatic epilepsy.

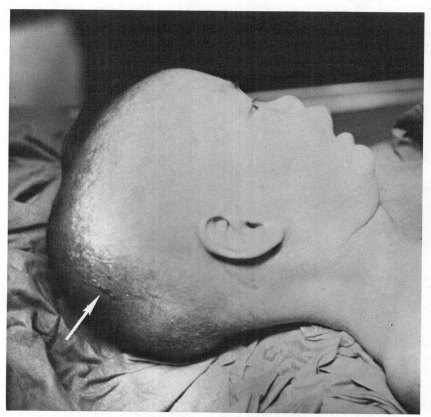

Figure 4-1 A seven-year-old male who sustained a fragment wound of the head (arrow) from an 82-mm mortar attack on his village.

---

*M.E. Carey, personal communication.

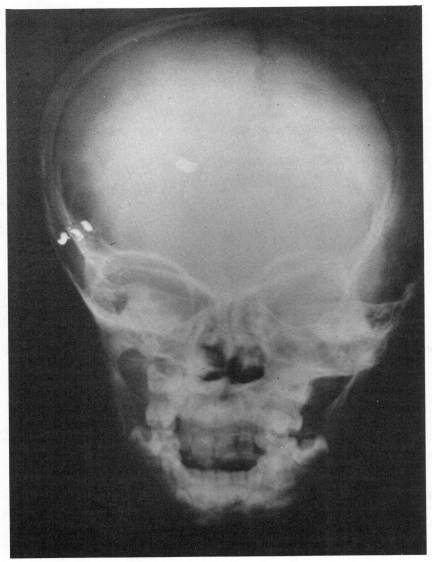

Figure 4-2 A skull radiogram in the A-P position reveals multiple metallic fragments along the right temporal region, as well as one near the midline.

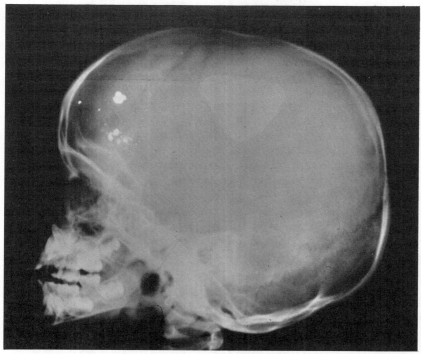

Figure 4-3 A lateral skull film confirms that at least the one large fragment is within the cranial cavity and thus provides indication for craniectomy and debridement.

A careful neurologic examination is essential to determine the extent of the intracranial damage and the localization of intracranial hematoma formation. The latter is facilitated by such noninvasive techniques as brain scan and computerized axial tomography, and where these are not possible, by the more hazardous invasive technique of carotid arteriography. Emergency burr holes are indicated in occipital, midparietal, and subtemporal regions if neurologic function deteriorates. Systemic arterial hypertension, widening of the pulse pressure, bradycardia, and declining respiratory rate suggest progressive increase in intracranial pressure and the possibility of compression or herniation of the medulla. Such signs as postauricular ecchymosis (Battle sign), and cerebrospinal fluid otorrhea or rhinorrhea also suggest a basilar skull fracture. The patient himself, if carefully questioned, can detect rhinorrhea by the taste of the glucose in the cerebrospinal fluid.

For obvious reasons, metallic fragments located deep within the substance of the brain, such as within the midbrain or thalamus, are usually not amenable to removal through neurosurgical craniectomy.

The trauma surgeon usually has not had sufficient training in neurosurgery to lead to the likelihood of performing a successful craniectomy; nonetheless, the trauma surgeon might well be called upon to perform burr holes for the urgent relief of dangerously increasing intracranial pressure. This relatively simple procedure may be lifesaving, and can be accomplished quickly and often without anesthesia. It should be within the capability of the surgeon who expects to undertake the primary care of trauma.

In the absence of immediate neurosurgical assistance and perhaps in preparation for neurosurgical intervention, several pharmacologic agents are effective against increased intracranial pressure, whether due to penetrating injuries such as gunshot wounds or, in fact, even to closed head injury. These include osmotic diuretics such as mannitol intravenously and renal tubular diuretics such as furosemide and ethacrynic acid. Diuresis probably is accompanied by reduction of both intravascular and interstitial volumes in the cranial cavity, relieving intracranial pressure and "buying time" for definitive neurosurgery. Corticosteroids in high dose (methylprednisolone—30 mg per kg, dexamethasone—6 mg per kg, or hydrocortisone—30 mg per kg, given intravenously) have been found effective in reducing edema of the brain in closed or penetrating head wounds. These agents may be administered prior to neurosurgery and certainly are indicated should neurosurgical intervention not be immediately available. In the latter case the dose and time of administration must be properly passed on to the neurosurgical team.

Since there is as yet no surgical repair of lacerated and contused brain tissue, prognosis is very grave for recovery and even survival when damage is extensive.

The Eye

The definitive management of penetrating wounds of the eye (Figures 4-4–4-6) belongs to the ophthalmologist. Primary treatment may be limited to an eye patch to minimize eye movement, discourage secondary infection, and comfort the patient. Complete loss of vision within the injured eye indicates evisceration or enucleation. Evisceration consists of removal of all of the scleral contents including the confines of the anterior and posterior chambers through an incision in the sclera at the limbus. This procedure leaves the ocular muscles intact and insures a better cosmetic result when a prosthesis is placed within the remaining sclera. Because this procedure carries a higher risk of sympathetic ophthalmia, enucleation is more commonly utilized.[21] Enucleation consists of removal of the orbital contents with the exception of the ocular muscles, which are sutured to a prosthesis, therefore, generally resulting in a less satisfactory cosmetic result than evisceration.

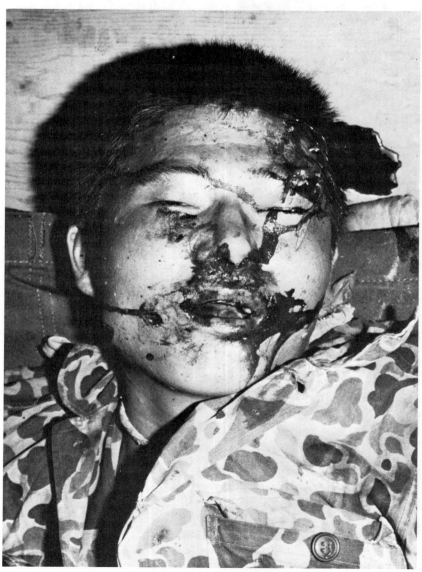

Figure 4-4　A 26-year-old man who sustained multiple fragment wounds from an 82-mm mortar attack.

40

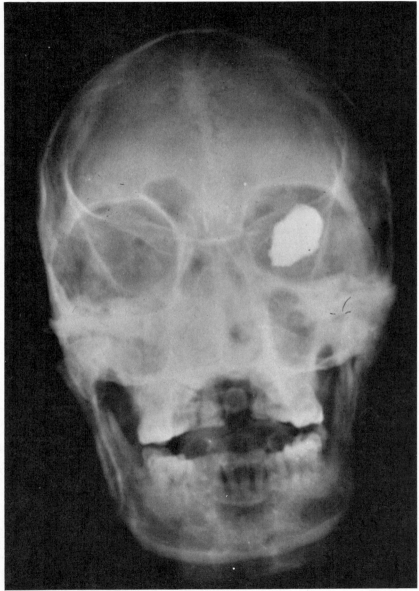

Figure 4-5 A skull radiogram (A-P) reveals a large metallic density in the region of the left orbit.

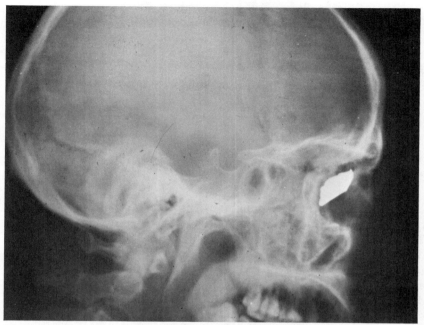

Figure 4-6 A lateral film confirms the presence of this fragment within the left orbit. This finding alone indicates the strong probability that the eye is not salvageable. The left eye was enucleated.

Urgency in the decision as to which operative procedure, if either, to pursue, or whether to attempt extraction of metallic fragments within the globe[22] in the hope of preserving visual function relates to the problem of sympathetic ophthalmia. This condition,[23,24] an apparent autoimmune uveitis of the uninvolved contralateral eye following within days or even years after a penetrating injury of the eye,[21] is an uncommon but extremely serious complication since it often leads to total blindness. It is reported to occur in 3% to 5% of penetrating eye injuries and in 80% of such cases it appears within three months of the initial injury.[24] Immunosuppressive drugs such as corticosteroids,[21,24] methotrexate, and azathioprine,[21] apparently have been effective in both the surgical and nonsurgical treatment of penetrating ocular injuries. Despite its infrequency, sympathetic ophthalmia is such a dire consequence that it must be considered in every penetrating eye injury, and the decision must be made as to whether the eye originally injured shows any likelihood of regaining useful vision. If it does not, enucleation or evisceration should be prompt. After sympathetic ophthalmia develops, these procedures may or may not be effective.[24]

Regardless of the operative procedure chosen, evisceration or enucleation, it is of paramount importance to remove all uveal tissue,[24] and probably for this reason enucleation is the more commonly utilized procedure. Here again, the trauma surgeon is advised to become familiar with this relatively simple ophthalmologic procedure since he may at some time be isolated from consultation with an ophthalmologist for more than several days.

The Ear

Blast injuries to the head include contusion and rupture of the tympanic membrane and dislocation of the ossicles within the middle ear. These and more serious injuries to the middle ear will, of course, diminish hearing on the injured side. Contusion of the tympanic membrane may be revealed otoscopically by engorged vessels, hemorrhage, and edema. Transudate or hemorrhage in the middle-ear cavity may distend the tympanic membrane. Bleeding into the external auditory canal may be from rupture of the membrane or fracture of the base of the skull. Both contusion and rupture of the tympanic membrane can be expected to resolve spontaneously. More serious injury may require reconstruction. In the interim, treatment is usually best limited to assessing the continuance and type of drainage within the external canal with a very loose cotton pack, and to discouraging infection by administering antibiotics systemically.

The Maxillofacial Area

Maxillofacial injuries primarily threaten the patient's life through hemorrhage and obstruction of his airway. The surgeon should be alerted to the need for a tracheostomy, which may be needed anyway for definitive surgical management. A surprisingly large percentage of patients who sustain gunshot wounds of the maxillofacial area (Figures 4-7-4-10) do, in fact, survive simply because very few vital organs except the airway are likely to be compromised. If the patient's vital signs are stable and normal and the airway clear, the surgeon should examine the maxilla, both externally and orally, as well as the bones articulating with it—the zygomatic, frontal, lacrimal, palatine, and ethmoid bones.

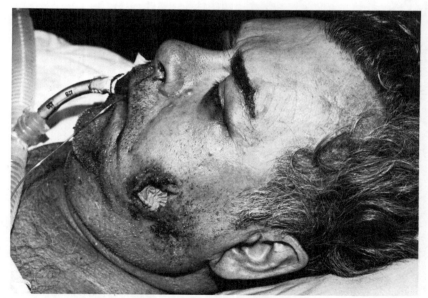

Figure 4-7 A 56-year-old, white male who sustained a 38-caliber (revolver) gunshot wound of the left side of the face at an immediate range. The wound of entrance has been packed, and an endotracheal tube is in position.

44

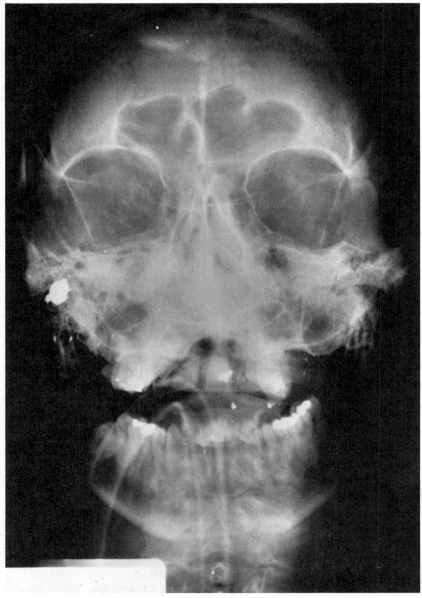

Figure 4-8 A skull radiogram (A-P view) reveals a large metallic fragment located in the region of the right antrum. Smaller metallic fragments are also seen.

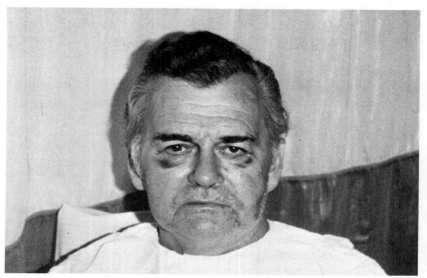

Figure 4-9 One week after injury, the patient exhibits only bilateral perior-bital ecchymosis. He survived without any significant maxillofacial surgery, but almost succumbed because attendants failed to address the urgent need to establish an airway.

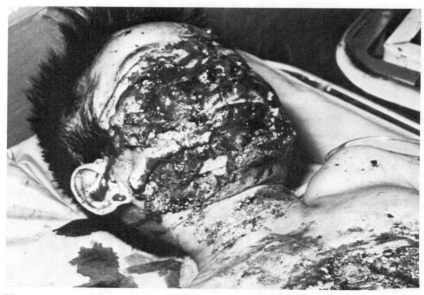

Figure 4-10 This eight-year-old boy sustained multiple fragment wounds from a detonated booby trap. He was dyspneic and had exposed mandible and maxilla, and not seen in these pictures, traumatic amputation of both hands, and evisceration of both liver and lung. He was declared expectant and died within six hours of reception. Had attempts been made to save this patient tracheostomy would have been necessary.

A blowout fracture of the maxilla can be identified by careful palpation of the inferior rim of the orbit, as well as a search for visual disturbance secondary to weakness of a prolapsed orbital muscle, secondary to the fracture of the floor of the orbit. Diplopia is strong evidence of a blowout fracture of the orbit and is secondary to displacement of the origin of the inferior oblique muscle. The injury may be accompanied by lancinating pain over the distribution of the zygomaticofacial, zygomaticotemporal, or infraorbital nerves. A defect in the floor of the orbit is relatively easily repaired surgically by inserting an acrylic prosthesis beneath the globe via an infraorbital skin incision.

Le Fort classified maxillofacial injuries[25] into three groups: (1) fracture of the maxilla (Figure 4-11), (2) fractures of both maxilla and nasal bones (Figure 4-12), and (3) fractures of maxilla, nasal bones, and maxillary sinuses (Figure 4-13). These injuries can be identified by a careful search with the gloved hand within and without the oral cavity for false motion, pain on motion, or tenderness during palpation of these bones.[26] The trauma surgeon will not likely be called upon for definitive care of these injuries which require external fixation utilizing suspension to the zygoma or skull. Nonetheless, he should be aware of the classification, diagnosis, and treatment of such injuries.

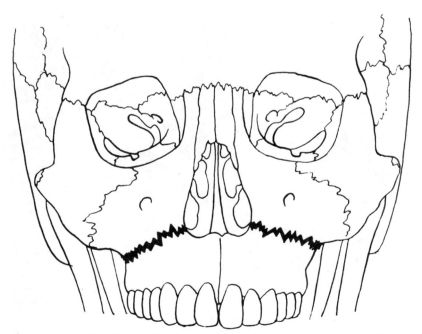

Figure 4-11 The Class I Le Fort maxillary fracture passes below the nasal bones. Figures 4-10, 4-11, and 4-12 reproduced by permission of the publisher, from T.J. Zaydon, and J.B. Brown, *Early Treatment of Facial Injuries.* Philadelphia: Lea & Febiger, 1964.

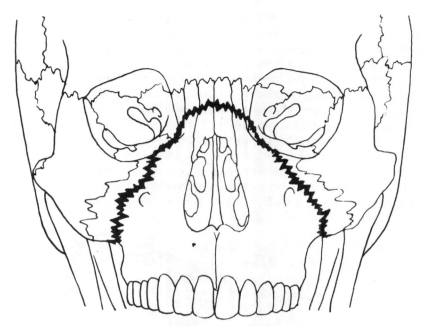

Figure 4-12 The Class II Le Fort maxillary fracture transsects the nasal bones.

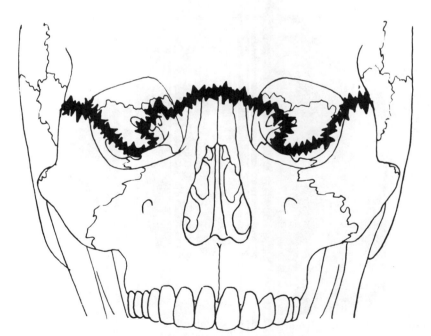

Figure 4-13 The Class III Le Fort maxillary fracture includes the zygoma and the frontal and ethmoyd bones.

Injuries to the mandible are usually evident from gross inspection. Because of their density and hardness, teeth can become impressive secondary missiles when struck by a bullet.[26] This phenomenon makes radiograms of the head even more important in the management of gunshot wounds. Definitive management of a mandibular fracture is usually beyond the capability of the trauma surgeon. Sometimes, however, he may not be able to obtain special help promptly. In such cases he is advised to stabilize the fractured mandible by maxillary fixation. This is a relatively routine maxillofacial procedure and consists of wiring together the teeth of the upper and lower jaws.

It is important to remember that maxillofacial injuries can be the cause of torrential hemorrhage, best controlled by ligation of the external carotid artery (Figures 4-14, 4-15). This can be accomplished readily

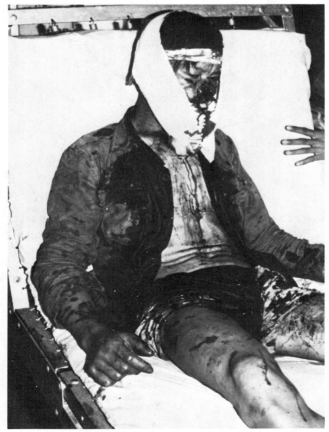

Figure 4-14 This 23-year-old man sustained an M-2 (38-caliber) carbine wound of the face. He arrived at the hospital two hours following wounding. He is in the sitting position because he encountered difficulty breathing when the nurse (hand) attempted to supinate him.

through an incision over the anterior border of the sternocleidomastoid muscle, identifying the common carotid artery and its bifurcation, so as to prevent accidental ligation of an internal carotid artery. The latter, of course, may be disastrous. Both external carotid arteries can be ligated, if necessary. Ischemic necrosis of the tip of the nose is an infrequent complication of bilateral ligation of the external carotid arteries, but this is a small price to pay for preventing fatal hemorrhage.

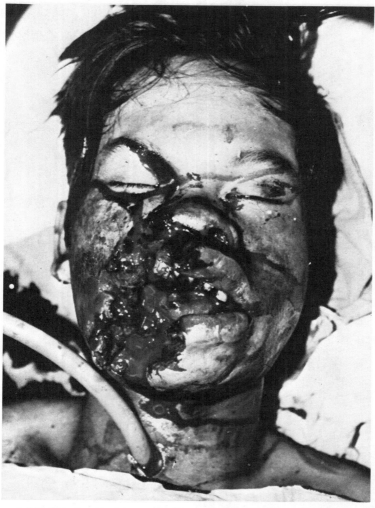

Figure 4-15 Tracheostomy was performed in the upright position to establish an airway so as to permit general anesthesia. At that point, the head dressing could be removed and the extent of the injury assessed. Extensive damage to both maxilla and mandible is apparent. Radiograms were not taken preoperatively because the patient's critical airway problem did not allow time.

50

Again, minimal debridement and careful reapproximation of all apparently partially avulsed tissues, including skin and muscle, will minimize the cosmetic loss attending maxillofacial injuries and such repair is usually well tolerated by victims of a gunshot wound of the face (Figures 4-16, 4-17).

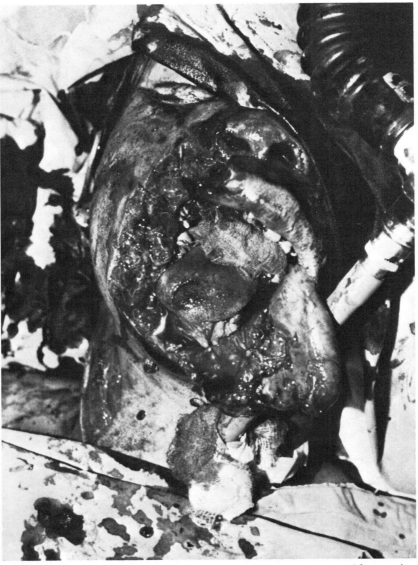

Figure 4-16 Debridement is carried out; the right common carotid artery has been exposed via the usual incision along the anterior border of the right sterno-cleidomastoid muscle, and the external carotid artery has been ligated.

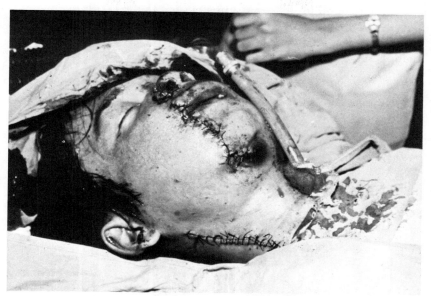

Figure 4-17 The facial debridement is followed with primary closure of all wounds, including the neck incision. These areas are empirically amenable to debridement and primary closure, whereas most other anatomic locations require delayed primary closure.

If the tongue is injured, its base should be surgically restored with suture reattachment of the frenulum linguae to prevent accidental obstruction of the oropharynx and asphyxiation. Such a procedure is superfluous if tracheostomy has been or is to be performed. As in other injuries to bony structures, loose, apparently nonviable fragments of bone probably should be removed in the process of debridement, although this principle is not without controversy.

A patient with a gunshot wound of the maxillofacial region often will not tolerate the supine position because of airway obstruction secondary to lacerated and edematous tissue or blood. This intolerance hinders oral intubation and standard endotracheal anesthesia. Therefore, a patient with a gunshot wound who is admitted to the emergency room with a head dressing (Figure 4-14), following resuscitation in the field, probably should proceed directly to the operating room. There, adequate lighting and surgical equipment will facilitate tracheostomy, which may in fact need to be performed with the patient in the upright position. Most facial gunshot wounds will require tracheostomy.[27] Necessary radiograms of the skull may have to be performed postoperatively.

Penetrating, as well as blunt injuries to the head and particularly to the face and eyes can seriously threaten the patient psychologically.

The physician and his assistants must attend to the resulting anxiety. Every effort should be made to reassure the patient that immediate, as well as late, reconstructive procedures usually result in restoration of function and a satisfactory cosmetic result (Figure 4-18).

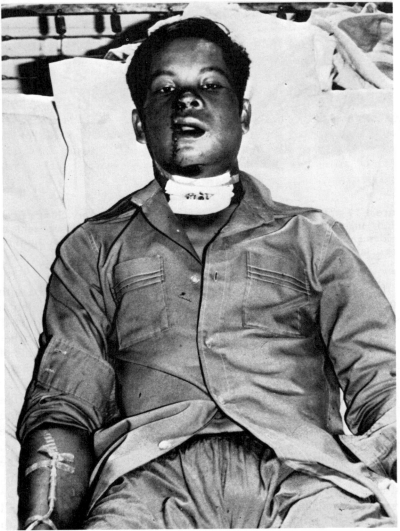

Figure 4-18   On the day following surgery, the patient is progressing satisfactorily with a tracheostomy tube in place. He is tolerating clear fluids by mouth and will now undergo appropriate radiographic investigation of the extent of maxillofacial injury in anticipation of planned reconstruction of fractures to these bones. A radiographic search for the possible presence of an intracranial metallic foreign body will be made simultaneously. Cosmetically, the result is at this point satisfactory.

SUMMARY

A gunshot wound of the head poses a serious problem for both patient and attendant. If brain is involved, survival is unpredictable; if another organ is injured, its future function will be problematic. The airway may be seriously threatened.

Missile damage is maximal because the abundance of bone and the presence of teeth provide the greatest potential for dissipation of kinetic energy. Radiograms of the head are critical determinants of management after assessment of neurologic and special organ (i.e., eye) function. Metallic foreign bodies within the skull indicate neurosurgical craniectomy and debridement in general. Resultant craniocerebral wounds require debridement and elevation of attendant depressed skull fractures. The presence of a metallic fragment within the brain stem is probably beyond the technical expertise of the neurosurgeon at present. Failure to debride such wounds, however, portends subsequent brain abscess and seizure disorder, since intracranial foreign body, other than just metal, is implied.

When head injury includes only maxillofacial damage, concern for adequacy of airway takes precedence. Tracheostomy is usually indicated and should be prompt. Fractures of mandible and maxilla need to be identified and stabilized with bony fixation.

Search for a blowout fracture of the orbit is indicated and readily treated. Diplopia is indicative. If the eye is involved in a gunshot wound of the head, vision determines treatment. Its presence suggests conservatism. Sympathetic ophthalmia is a realistic, albeit infrequent, complication of attempts to preserve an injured eye. If vision is seriously compromised, or absent, following orbital gunshot, then enucleation is indicated. Evisceration is a lesser, more cosmetically acceptable, but more hazardous alternative.

A principle of head wounds is that debridement and primary closure is indicated. The head tolerates this approach; it is cosmetically more critical, and it has been successful empirically. If hemorrhage is difficult to control, then ligation of one or both external carotid arteries is useful. The latter procedure demands formal neck exploration to ascertain that the external, and not internal, carotid artery is ligated. Both external carotid arteries can be ligated if necessary. A complication of the latter is loss of the tip of the nose due to ischemia.

REFERENCES

1. Lattimer, J.K. The wound that killed Lincoln. *JAMA.* 187:480–489, 1964.

2. Lattimer, J.K., Lattimer, J., and Lattimer, G. An experimental study of the backward movement of President Kennedy's head. *Surg Gynecol Obstet.* 142:246–254, 1976.

3. Maughon, J.S. An inquiry into the nature of wounds resulting in killed in action in Vietnam. *Milit Med.* 135:8-13, 1970.

4. Cushing, H. A study of a series of wounds involving the brain and its enveloping structures. *Br J Surg.* 5:558-684, 1918.

5. Gurdjian, E.S. The treatment of penetrating wounds of the brain sustained in warfare: a historical review. *J Neurosurg.* 39:157-167, 1974.

6. Small, J.M., and Turner, E.A. A surgical experience of 1200 cases of penetrating brain wounds in battle, N.W. Europe, 1944-45. *Br J Surg.* War Surg Suppl 1, pp. 62-74, 1947.

7. Matson, D.D., and Wolkin, J. Hematomas associated with penetrating wounds of the brain. *J Neurosurg.* 3:46-53, 1946.

8. Wallace, P.B., and Meirowsky, A.M. The repair of dural defects by graft: an analysis of 540 penetrating wounds of the brain incurred in the Korean War. *Ann Surg.* 151:174-180, 1960.

9. Schorstein, J. Intracranial haematoma in missile wounds. *Br J Surg.* War Surg Suppl 1, pp. 96-111, 1947.

10. Barnett, J.C., and Meirowsky, A.M. Intracranial hematomas associated with penetrating wounds of the brain. *J Neurosurg.* 12:34-38, 1955.

11. Lewin, W., and Gibson, R.M. Missile head wounds in the Korean campaign: a survey of British casualties. *Br J Surg.* 43:628-632, 1956.

12. Meirowsky, A.M. Penetrating craniocerebral trauma: observations in Korean War. *JAMA.* 154:666-669, 1954.

13. Hammon, W.M. Analysis of 2187 consecutive penetrating wounds of the brain from Vietnam. *J Neurosurg.* 34:127-131, 1971.

14. Mathews, W.E. The early treatment of craniocerebral missile injuries: experience with 92 cases. *J Trauma.* 12:939-954, 1972.

15. Carey, M.E. Young, H.F., and Mathis, J.L. The neurosurgical treatment of craniocerebral missile wounds in Vietnam. *Surg Gynecol Obstet.* 135:386-390, 1972.

16. Raimondi, A.J., and Samuelson, G.H. Craniocerebral gunshot wounds in civilian practice. *J Neurosurg.* 32:647-653, 1970.

17. Hubschmann, O., Shapiro, K., Baden, M. et al. Craniocerebral gunshot injuries in civilian practice-prognostic criteria and surgical management: experience with 82 cases. *J Trauma.* 19:6-12, 1979.

18. Gerber, A.M., and Moody, R.A. Craniocerebral missile injuries in the monkey: an experimental physiological model. *J Neurosurg.* 36:43-49, 1972.

19. Freytag, E. Autopsy findings in head injuries from firearms: statistical evaluation of 254 cases. *Arch Pathol.* 76:215-225, 1963.

20. Gurdjian, E.S., and Gurdjian, E.S. Acute head injuries. Collective reviews. *Surg Gynecol Obstet.* 146:805-820, 1978.

21. Makley, T.A., and Azar, A. Sympathetic ophthalmia: a long-term follow-up. *Arch Ophthalmol.* 96:257-262, 1978.

22. Mandelcorn, M.S., and Brown, M. Computed axial tomography localization of intra-orbital foreign body. *Can J Ophthalmol.* 13:213-215, 1978.

23. Lewis, M.L., Gass, D.M., and Spencer, W.H. Sympathetic uveitis after trauma and vitrectomy. *Arch Ophthalmol.* 96:263-267, 1978.

24. Paton, D., and Goldberg, M.F. *Management of Ocular Injuries.* Philadelphia: W.B. Saunders Co., 1976.

25. Le Fort, R. Étude expérimentale sur les fractures de la mâchoire supérieure. *Rev Chir.* 23:208, 1901.

26. Cruse, C.W., Blevins, P.K., and Luce, E.A. Naso-ethmoid orbital fractures. *J Trauma.* (In press). Presented at the 39th Annual Meeting of the American Association for the Surgery of Trauma. Chicago, September 13-15, 1979.

27. Shuck, L.W., Orgel, M.G., and Vogel, A.V. Self-inflicted gunshot wounds to the face: a review of 15 cases. *J Trauma*. (In press). Presented at the 39th Annual Meeting of the American Association for the Surgery of Trauma. Chicago, September 13–15, 1979.

5 The Neck

If hemorrhage exists from injury to a large vessel, it must of course receive the surgeon's first and most earnest care. He should not trust to the pressure of a tourniquet, but secure it at once by ligature. Without this safeguard during the transport, and while in the hands of uneducated attendants, the life of the wounded man might be endangered, either from debility consequent upon gradual loss of blood or from sudden fatal hemorrhage. It has been recommended by some surgeons that all attendants whose duties consist in carrying the wounded from a field of battle should be directed, when bleeding is observed, to *place a finger in the wound, and keep it there during the transport* until the aid of a surgeon is obtained. The precise spot where compression by the finger is wanted, and the degree of pressure necessary, will be quickly made manifest to the sight by the effects on the flow of blood. Such a practice seems to offer less objection than the use of tourniquets by men whose knowledge of their proper application must be exceedingly limited.*

*Longmore, T. *Gunshot Wounds.* Philadelphia: J.B. Lippincott Co., 1863.

The increasing frequency with which firearms are becoming the instruments of assault in American civil life is strikingly evident in the case of wounds of the neck. Gunshot wounds of this region have now become more common than knife wounds.[1-8] When this relative frequency is coupled with the fact that the mortality rate from gunshot wounds (10%)[1-6] of the neck is currently five times that of knife wounds (2%)[2-9] the problem of gunshot wounds of the neck assumes substantial proportions.

Almost all gunshot wounds of the neck are penetrating when "penetrating" is defined as passing through the platysma muscle, or in other regions of the neck going deeper than the subcutaneous tissue.

In both types of wounds, controversy exists as to whether all penetrating wounds of the neck should be explored,[10-12] and whether or not there is evidence preoperatively of injury to major structures.[4,5] In favor of exploration is the report that the incidence of preoperatively unrecognized major structural injury may run as high as 33%,[3] and the experience of very low mortality (less than 1%) and morbidity (approximately 1%) from surgical exploration.[1,2,4,5] The conservative argument is that exploration should be reserved for cases in which injury to major structures, especially the carotid arteries, the esophagus, and the airway is suspected. It is supported by results in several large series[9,13,14] in which more than half the patients were treated conservatively, and of these, only 2% subsequently required surgery. Since World War II, mandatory surgical exploration for all penetrating wounds of the neck has, however, been gaining favor.

The neck was the site of fatal high velocity missile wounds in 5% of the cases in the Korean War[15] and about 7% in the Vietnam War.[16] Compared to these frequencies, the abdomen was the site of fatal injuries in 9% and 10% of cases respectively, for these two wars.[15,16] Thus, despite its relatively small size, the neck is frequently the site of fatal wounds.

The most critical cervical structures are, of course, the spine and spinal cord, the esophagus, the trachea and larynx, the common and internal carotid arteries, and the internal jugular veins. Injury to any of these carries an immediate threat to life and must be recognized and repaired, or managed so as to minimize this threat, or minimize lasting disability. Injuries to other cervical structures, with the exception of the very uncommon bilateral severance of the vagus nerves, do not usually pose an immediate threat to life and do not require immediate surgical intervention.

The foremost consideration in gunshot wounds of the neck is the possibility of cervical spinal cord injury. Hemorrhage and respiratory obstruction should not distract those in initial attendance from this concern and the concern that by their manipulations they may make such injury worse. Rotation of the head on the neck, or the neck on the thorax, and the flexion of either the head or neck, must be avoided until such injury, or potential injury, seems improbable.

The apparent path of the bullet, the presence or absence of pain and tenderness over the cervical spine, the persistence of respiratory movements, and of motility and sensation in the extremities can be quickly ascertained while attending to other life-threatening conditions. If vertebral or spinal cord injury is suspected, the patient must not be transported before immobilizing the head with sandbags or similar pads. When other threats to life such as hemorrhage and respiratory obstruction have been met, a limited but precise neurologic examination is indicated if injury to the cervical spine or spinal cord seems probable. If spinal injury is suspected, the patient should not be transported except on a spinal board or its equivalent. The head must be immobilized with respect to the board with adhesive tape to the forehead for example.

Once in a medical facility, a lateral radiogram of the cervical spine will be diagnostic. The radiogram should be made with the shoulders depressed to facilitate viewing the C7-T1 interspace. Unless the resuscitation table is equipped with an x-ray cassette holder, the A-P film is contraindicated, as this would require flexing the neck.

If cervical spine or spinal cord injury is diagnosed or suspected, skeletal traction should be instituted with two-point fixation on the calvarium. Countertraction is provided by placing the rest of the body in slight dependency. If there is progression of neurologic signs and evidence that the cord is not completely transsected, surgical decompression through cervical laminectomy should be considered. This decision, however, requires the most exquisite neurosurgical judgment. A so-called "mini myelogram" through the C1-C2 interspace has been an advocated step in the emergent diagnosis of acute cord injury where doubt exists.[17]

THE CAROTID ARTERIES

Few events are more tragic than the preventable exsanguination of a previously healthy person after an injury to a major vessel. In the crucial few minutes, friends, relatives, even professionals and those trained in first aid, stand immobile or undertake ineffective measures. The following three examples of hemorrhage from a carotid artery or a major branch are typical of many such occurrences in civil life today.

> On June 7, 1979, a five-year-old boy was attacked by a leopard at a circus in front of hundreds of onlookers, and bitten in the neck. He was pronounced dead 90 minutes later. The cause of death was exsanguination; autopsy revealed an injured occipital artery.

On May 25, 1976, a 14-year-old high school student was cut by flying glass resulting from a firecracker prank, in the presence of classmates and a teacher. She was DOA at the local hospital 30 minutes later. Death was from exsanguination. Autopsy revealed a lacerated carotid artery.

On May 20, 1974, a 27-year-old man was slashed by a razor blade in an argument over a dog. While six friends watched, he exsanguinated within minutes in broad daylight. Autopsy revealed a severed carotid artery.

Details of these cases are found in the Appendix.

In each of the cases cited above, immediate application of an index finger directly and forcibly into the source of the jet of blood would have arrested the hemorrhage and saved the life, probably without ischemic damage to the brain. Such pressure *must be maintained* until definitive surgical control is instituted, i.e., in the operating room.

Because of their linear extent in the neck, the carotid arteries are injured relatively frequently in gunshot wounds and other penetrating injuries of the neck. The common carotid arteries are the arteries most frequently injured.[1,4,5,12,13] A hematoma is usually, but not always, indication that an artery rather than a jugular vein has been lacerated. Although hematoma is occasionally seen following internal jugular venous injury, usually the pressures within that vessel are insufficient to generate a cervical hematoma against the resistance of the carotid sheath.

A carotid arterial injury will occasionally be identified by the absence of a pulse in the superficial temporal or facial artery. Thus, the physical examination should include palpation of these pulses.

A more sophisticated assessment of the pulse distal to a suspected arterial injury involves use of the Doppler principle,[18] which is a sonic translation of blood flow. Doppler pulse-recording devices are commercially available in pocket size. Directional Doppler pulse recording is a further sophistication of this technique and is especially applicable to evaluating the integrity of arteries of the head and neck, since it can determine the presence of collateral blood flow from the contralateral carotid arterial system. The latter implies resistance to flow through the ipsilateral, presumably injured, side. Ultimately, angiography may prove necessary to identify possible intracranial internal carotid arterial injuries.[1]

A suspected carotid arterial injury should alert the surgical team to prepare the patient so as to have ready access to a saphenous vein autograft, should the defect be of sufficient size to preclude primary anastomosis. Considering the time required to gain control of the carotid arterial injury through the neck exploration, and the time required to remove a sufficient segment of saphenous vein as well as to prepare it for autografting, it is quite appropriate for a second operative team to proceed immediately with removal of the venous autograft while the other team explores the neck. Unnecessary resection of a segment of saphenous vein is acceptable if the object is to minimize the time of carotid arterial occlusion. This is particularly true if suitable catheters for internal shunting of the carotid artery are not available. Although a number of approaches to neck exploration are available to the surgeon, those most commonly utilized are an oblique incision along the anterior border of the sternocleidomastoid muscle, or a transverse cervical incision midway between the prominence of the thyroid cartilage and the suprasternal notch. The patient should, of course, be positioned with the head extended and the shoulders elevated.

Patients with carotid arterial injuries can be divided into two groups: (1) those who are neurologically intact, and (2) those who are neurologically compromised.[11] Signs and symptoms in the latter group of patients may simulate those characteristic of a cerebrovascular accident. Hypertension and bradycardia may be present; the patient may be obtunded; the ipsilateral pupil is often dilated and fixed, and there is evidence of long tract signs, characteristically, a contralateral hemiparesis and hemisensory defect. Disparity of reflexes, including hyperreflexia and pathologic reflexes on the contralateral side, are also seen acutely following carotid arterial injury. In this latter group of patients, although surgery is mandatory to control the defect in the carotid artery, the procedure of choice is ligation, proximally and distally, since reconstruction, in the face of a fixed neurologic defect, may result in the conversion of an ischemic, or "white" infarct of the brain into a hemorrhagic, or "red," infarct.[11] The latter phenomenon augments the increased intracranial pressure, due to the resulting edema of the brain, and can convert an otherwise salvageable, although neurogically compromised, patient to one characterized by rapid deterioration, as a result of further brain-stem herniation.

In the group of patients who are neurologically intact, the arterial injury is managed in the usual fashion after gaining control of blood flow proximal and distal to the vascular injury (Figures 5-1–5-6). Almost invariably, healthy individuals will tolerate cross-clamping of a common or internal carotid artery for the purpose of immediate vascular repair.[19] However, especially in older individuals it is safer to ascertain whether there is sufficient collateral flow to the brain through the vertebral and/or contralateral arteries by measuring "stump pressure" or "back pressure" immediately upon occluding the artery cephalad to the injury. If the pressure in the clamped distal stump, as recorded through a needle inserted into this stump, exceeds 50 mm Hg, collateral flow may be assumed sufficient to permit continuing proximal occlusion in order to accomplish the repair. In case a manometer is not available to the surgeon, so-called *field stump pressure* can be measured. This latter procedure is accomplished by releasing the distal clamp while maintaining occlusion of that portion of the common carotid artery proximal to the injury. If a vigorous jet of blood escapes from the wound the presumption is that there is adequate perfusion through the circle of Willis, from the opposite side, as well as through the ipsilateral vertebral artery. In fact, if the patient is properly positioned, the height of the column of blood can be measured with a centimeter rule. This height, in centimeters, divided by 1.3 (the approximate specific gravity of mercury), will give the exact pressure in mm Hg. The latter maneuver is recommended only for the more compulsive trauma surgeon!

If perfusion of the brain is insufficient as indicated by manometry, an internal shunt should be maintained during the repair. A variety of vascular shunts are manufactured specifically for carotid arterial surgery, but any flexible tubing of appropriate caliber will suffice in an emergency.

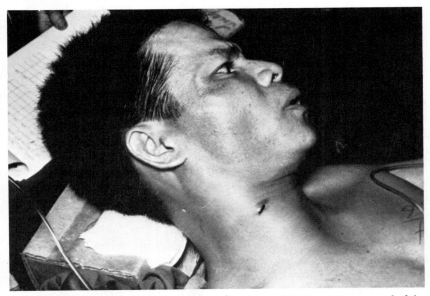

Figure 5-1   This 23-year-old soldier sustained an AK-47 gunshot wound of the neck. Aside from the small skin laceration involving the right side of the neck, the patient was asymptomatic, and physical exam was unremarkable.

Courtesy of U.S. Army–Vietnam Surgical Trauma Collection, Armed Forces Institute of Pathology, Washington, DC.

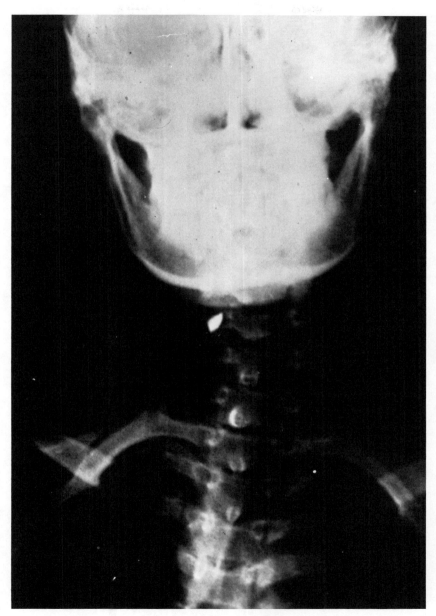

Figure 5-2 A neck radiogram reveals a metallic foreign body in the region of the right paraspinal area at the level of C3.

Courtesy of U.S. Army–Vietnam Surgical Trauma Collection, Armed Forces Institute of Pathology, Washington, DC.

64

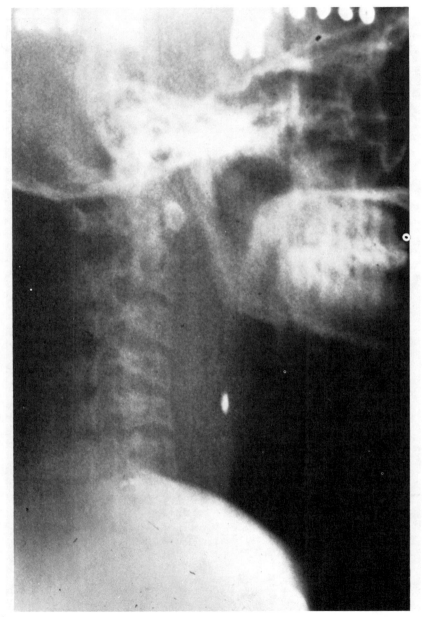

Figure 5-3 A lateral radiogram of the neck reveals the fragment to be located anterior to the cervical spine.

Courtesy of U.S. Army–Vietnam Surgical Trauma Collection, Armed Forces Institute of Pathology, Wash:ngton, DC.

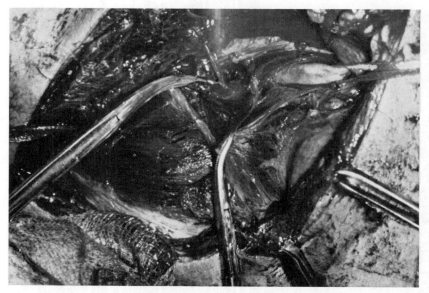

Figure 5-4 Neck exploration, via a standard oblique incision located over the anterior border of the right sternocleidomastoid muscle, revealed a defect in the common carotid artery. Proximal and distal control was accomplished with appropriately placed umbilical tapes. Release of the distal (cephalic) tape was associated with a vigorous jet of blood exiting the common carotid arterial defect. This so-called field stump pressure suggests that sufficient collateral circulation originates from the contralateral common carotid arterial and basilar arterial contributions to the circle of Willis to provide for adequate perfusion of the branches of the right internal carotid artery to allow cross-clamping of this vessel in order to effect appropriate repair.

Courtesy of U.S. Army–Vietnam Surgical Trauma Collection, Armed Forces Institute of Pathology, Washington, DC.

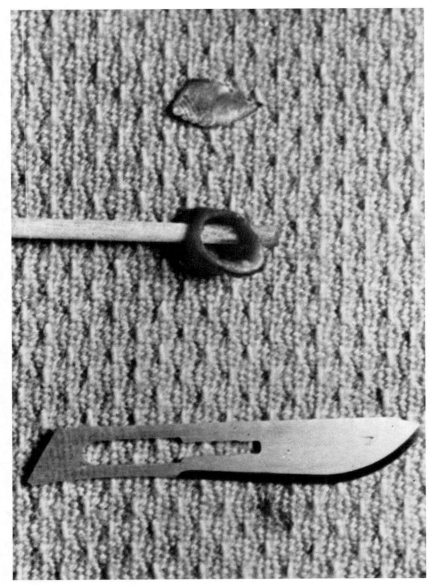

Figure 5-5 The resected injured common carotid arterial segment is exhibited along with the metallic fragment (a piece of copper jacketing from the AK-47 round) and a #10 Bard-Parker scalpel blade for size comparison. The applicator stick demonstrates the through-and-through nature of the common carotid arterial injury.

Courtesy of U.S. Army–Vietnam Surgical Trauma Collection, Armed Forces Institute of Pathology, Washington, DC.

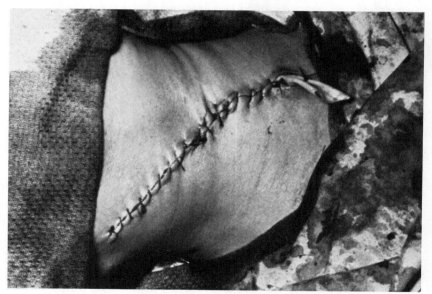

Figure 5-6 Primary anastomosis of the common carotid artery was accomplished and the neck wound was closed in layers, and a single Penrose drain positioned dependently to protect against possible missed esophageal injury.

Courtesy of U.S. Army–Vietnam Surgical Trauma Collection, Armed Forces Institute of Pathology, Washington, DC.

The common carotid artery and its branches, like other elastic arteries, are quite extensible, especially in younger people, who are the ones more frequently wounded by firearms. Such arteries can be readily stretched almost twofold. For this reason, mobilization proximally and distally will allow, in most cases, sufficient length of artery to permit adequate debridement and primary anastomosis. Debridement should extend one millimeter or more beyond the edges of the wound, since it is known that trauma to arteries is more extensive histologically than apparent grossly.[20] Anastomosis with 5–0, monofilamentous, atraumatic suture is the recommended technique of reapproximation. The size of the artery favors a continuous suture. If the defect is so great that primary anastomosis is not possible, then the material of choice is as mentioned—a reversed saphenous vein autograft.

The neck, like the head and external genitalia, can be debrided and closed primarily, unlike other parts of the body which must be closed secondarily. Nonetheless, a gunshot wound of the neck is considered a "dirty" wound, and for that reason, a cloth prosthesis is considered by most trauma surgeons to be contraindicated in the management of carotid arterial injuries. Some[8] disagree and advocate cloth prostheses in preference to autogenous saphenous vein in the management of vascular injuries if primary anastomosis is impossible and the wound is grossly contaminated. Lateral suture technique (i.e., closure of the vascular wound by continuous suture), can be employed if there is a partial and relatively simple laceration of the artery. Lateral suture technique frequently compromises the lumen. Most gunshot wounds of the carotid artery do not lend themselves to this form of surgical repair. Finally, a saphenous vein patch graft occasionally can be used effectively to close a defect in the carotid artery when there are reasons not to use other methods.

Care must be taken to prevent the passage of even a tiny bubble of air through the distal carotid artery following completion of the anastomosis and removal of the vascular clamps. This is best accomplished by removing the distal clamp first, and prior to securing the last one or two sutures in the anastomosis or arteriotomy closure. Anticoagulation is usually not necessary. The arteriotomy should be covered with muscle. A Penrose drain is placed before the neck incision is closed primarily.

Because the available length for repair of an injured internal carotid artery is quite limited, there is a tendency to accept ligation as definitive management, as an alternative to primary repair. Apparently, such ligation can be accomplished in most individuals under 30 years of age without neurologic complications.[1,5] However, arterial repair is preferable to ligation because a small percentage of those treated by ligation will develop neurologic damage, because this percentage increases with age, and because in later life such ligation may diminish the individual's tolerance to the development of atherosclerosis.

THE JUGULAR VEIN

When the neck wound may have included a laceration of the internal (or external) jugular vein, the danger from air embolus[6,21,22] and sudden death is real. Those in attendance, focusing upon the control of bleeding and contemplating venous repair, may forget that in the erect or sitting position, the pressure in the caudal end of the internal jugular vein tends to follow the alternating positive and negative pressures in the thorax. As the amplitude of these oscillations of pressure increases with exertion or anxiety, the danger of the entrance of air far exceeds the danger of loss of blood from a lacerated jugular vein. Conversely, in the supine position, under similar circumstances, bleeding attends such injuries rather than air embolization. As gentle local pressure controls bleeding, so does it control the entrance of air. An embolism is most unlikely if the patient is supine, for the reasons mentioned.

Because of the relative inelasticity and large diameter of the internal jugular vein, laceration is usually treated by ligation. Ligation of both internal jugular veins usually is tolerated, as the experience with bilateral radical neck dissection for cancer has shown. However, bilateral ligation may result in visual disturbance, headache, papilledema, oropharyngeal edema, and even death. Whenever possible, the internal jugular vein should be repaired. Repair of the external or anterior jugular veins is unnecessary.

Hyperventilation resulting from anxiety secondary to the injury and its initial management, as well as during ventilation accompanying induction of anesthesia, favors the introduction of air into an exposed internal jugular venous laceration. For this reason, it is of paramount importance that both surgeon and anesthesiologist recognize the potential threat and take appropriate precautions to prevent its occurrence.

Probably the most common technique for repairing an injured internal jugular vein is lateral suture, although the most common procedure is ligation. The former technique is likely to compromise the lumen and reduce flow. An alternative is use of spiral vein,[23] or compilation[24] grafts constructed from autogenous saphenous vein.

THE ESOPHAGUS

The esophagus is of paramount concern in management of penetrating injury of the neck. History and physical examination alone seldom

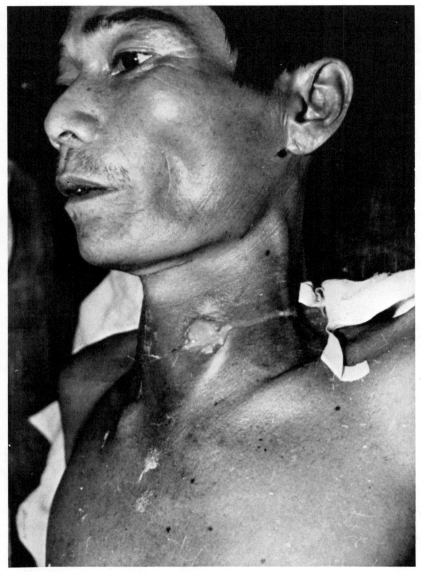

Figure 5-7 This 43-year-old farmer sustained multiple fragment wounds of the neck and abdomen when his village was struck by 82-mm mortars. He was treated with abdominal exploration, small-bowel resection, and diverting colostomy for related intraabdominal injuries. No therapy was directed to his neck wound. Ten days later, he was brought to the hospital because of fever and prostration. A foul-smelling discharge exits the neck wound. He is febrile, hypotensive, and exhibits tachycardia, tachypnea, and he is obtunded. Cellulitis and crepitation surround the neck wound.

provide the diagnosis, in contrast to injury to most other major cervical structures. Untreated, an injury penetrating the esophagus will almost invariably lead to fatal septicemia within 10 days (Figures 5-7–5-10).

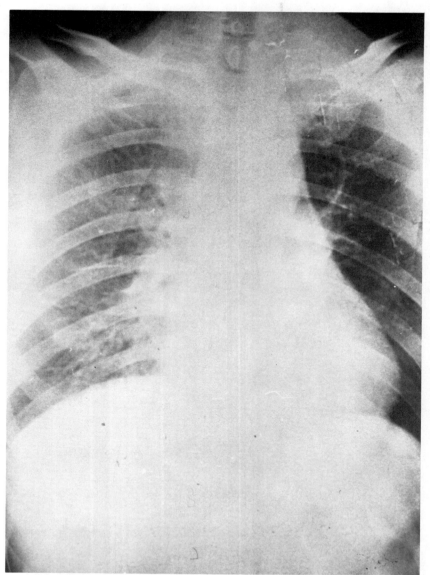

Figure 5-8 Chest radiogram (supine) reveals a decreased lucency to the right hemithorax and confirms auscultatory findings of decreased breath sounds on that side. No xiphisternal crunch (Hamman sign) or radiographic evidence of mediastinal air was documented. (Several small metalic foreign bodies are seen radiographically within the right side of the superior mediastinum.)

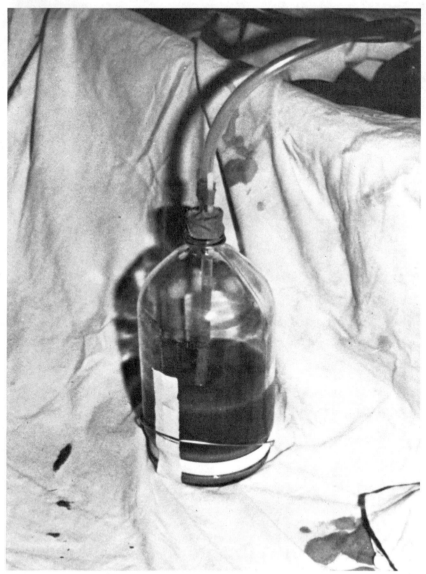

Figure 5-9 Right tube thoracostomy produced sanguinopurulent drainage which was foul smelling and indicated empyema.

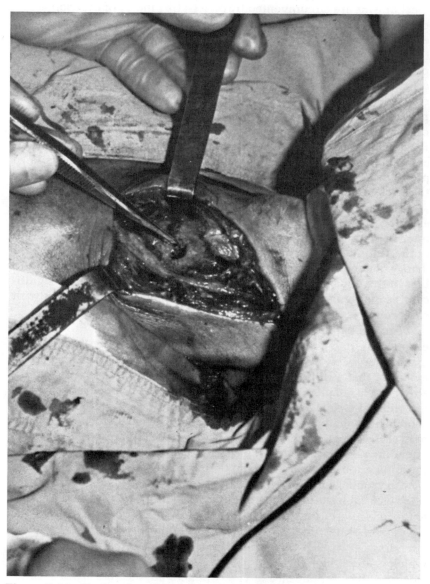

Figure 5-10 Exploration of the left neck revealed a large defect in the cervical esophagus, which was drained. The patient died within hours of surgery. The cause of death was sepsis secondary to mediastinitis and empyema, all the result of delayed treatment of an injury to the esophagus.

Normally, the esophageal mucosa with its barrier of stratified squamous epithelium, and the acid secretion of the stomach, are adequate barriers to invasion by swallowed bacteria. When these defense mechanisms are circumvented by penetrating injury of the esophagus, bacterially contaminated saliva and ingestants are extruded into the easily developed fascial spaces of the neck, particularly the one between the visceral and prevertebral deep fascial layers. By virtue of positive intraluminal pressure in the esophagus during swallowing and a mean negative pressure in the thorax, this fascial space is readily cleaved caudally through the neck, superior mediastinum, and posterior mediastinum, by contaminated saliva and ingestants, to induce mediastinitis. This rapidly progresses to bacteremia and to an extension into a pleural cavity, producing empyema and septicemia. This complication of a penetrating injury to the cervical esophagus is so probable as to justify surgical exploration for any penetrating injury to the neck, and insertion of a single Penrose drain.

The question of esophageal injury can be reliably resolved by esophagoscopy if the patient is undergoing general anesthesia for treatment of wounds of other regions, obviating the need for an exploration of the wound of the neck. We believe exploration of the neck is mandatory in penetrating neck injuries; however, exploration is not infallible. In the midst of extensive damage to cervical structures, a significant esophageal injury can be missed. Esophagoscopy together with exploration is probably optimal.

The appearance of blood within the esophagus may identify an esophageal injury that is otherwise unrecognized at the time of neck exploration. Conversely, negative esophagoscopy is good supporting evidence that significant injury to the esophagus has not occurred. In either event, exploration of the neck, viewing of the esophagus, and insertion of a single Penrose drain to be left in place for 10 days will establish an adequate sinus track that will prevent a morbid sequence of events. A greater awareness of the potential injury to the esophagus attending penetrating neck injuries has probably done more to reduce morbidity and mortality than any other single advance (Table 5-1).

An esophageal injury should be repaired primarily in layers, with a fine absorbable suture to the mucosa, and a fine nonabsorbable suture to the muscularis, each in interrupted fashion. For obvious reasons, the technique of repair plays a relatively minor role in the outcome attending cervical esophageal injuries. It is the drainage of the wound which is lifesaving, not the repair of the esophagus. Although primary closure of the esophageal tear is recommended, the defect would probably heal spontaneously with time. Following repair, gastric decompression should be instituted to prevent regurgitation of gastric contents into the cervical esophagus. Once normal gastric emptying is

Table 5-1
**Results of Surgical Management of Penetrating Neck Trauma
at a Large Urban Hospital Where Mandatory Neck Exploration
Was the Policy.**

Exploration	No.	Morbidity (%)	Mortality (%)
Positive* (37%)	90	8	9
Negative (63%)	156	1	0

Source: Saletta, J.D., Lowe, R.J., Lim, L.T. et al. Penetrating trauma of the neck. *J Trauma.* 16:579–587, 1976.
*14% unrecognized (preoperative), major, structural injury

ascertained in the postoperative period, oral intake may proceed beginning gradually with clear liquids. Strictures of the esophagus may result from esophageal injuries, during the late postoperative period, regardless of how carefully the repair is executed, but they should be amenable to dilation by bougies.

THE LARYNX AND TRACHEA

Gunshot injuries of the larynx and trachea are infrequently seen in emergency rooms. The reasons are two: (1) such injuries are usually associated with fatal exsanguination from injured common carotid arteries and internal jugular veins, and (2) airway obstruction is fatal before the patient reaches the hospital.

Signs of injury of airway in the neck include dyspnea, cyanosis, bubbling and foaming of the wound, dysphonia, stridor, and subcutaneous emphysema. The latter may extend to the face and/or the mediastinum. Mediastinal emphysema may be detected on the auscultation of the anterior thorax. Hamman sign,[25] a crunching sound on auscultation over the xiphisternum, is indicative of mediastinal emphysema, which may progress to cardiac tamponade (the signs of which are discussed in the next chapter).

In injuries of the larynx and trachea, as in injuries to the maxillofacial region, intubation through the pharynx may be difficult due to obstruction by damaged cartilage. Too much time should not be wasted in such attempts. Intubation can be adequately performed through the injured airway in the neck, or through a formal tracheostomy or cricothyroidotomy.

Management of injuries to the trachea and thyroid cartilage are based primarily on the location of the injury. If a small defect is identified below the thyroid cartilage it can be converted at the time of surgery, or even prior to surgery, into a tracheostomy, and its management during the postoperative period is much the same as that of any other tracheostomy for airway obstruction.[26] Large tears in the trachea, or rupture separations, require prompt surgical repair to restore the airway and prevent late sequelae such as stricture formation and stenosis. Proximal tracheostomy is usually needed to protect the tracheal repair. Injuries to the thyroid cartilage are best treated at the time of surgery with closure utilizing nonabsorbable suture; fine stainless steel wire is entirely appropriate. Injuries to the vocal folds may require splinting with plastic implants, and ultimately otolaryngologic reconstruction to restore phonation.[26] Overlooked or untreated injuries to the trachea will commonly present as respiratory distress due to ingrowth of granulation tissue within 7 to 10 days.[26]

MUSCLES AND TENDONS

The question often arises as to whether important skeletal muscles, ligaments, tendons, and components of the brachial plexus that are encountered during surgical management of neck wounds should be repaired primarily. Although the experience is that the neck tolerates debridement and primary closure better than the trunk and extremities (but perhaps less well than the face), cervical muscles, ligaments, and tendons are generally not repaired. In the case of the smaller muscles and tendons, functional loss from transsection is usually not serious. In the case of larger muscles, transsection is seldom complete in a salvageable patient. If it is, as for example in the case of the sternocleidomastoid muscle, the decision to repair or not depends upon the attention needed for more threatening associated injuries, and the extent of required debridement of muscle.

NERVES

When major cervical nerves, such as the superior or recurrent laryngeal,[27] spinal accessory, vagus, phrenic, sympathetic trunk, and other components of the cervical and brachial plexuses are injured by gunshot, they are seldom repaired. Repair is not attempted, either because the functional loss is readily compensated for (as in the case of the phrenic nerve[28]), because the extent of tissue damage and degree of contamination make successful repair unlikely, or because the distance between the nerve lesion and the effector organ innervated is so great (as in the case of lesions of the brachial plexus) that muscle atrophy is advanced before regenerating axons reach the effector organ.[29] When the function involved is critical (as in the case of a laryngeal nerve) and other aspects of the injury permit, repair should be attempted. Primary anastomosis at the time of injury can be expected to yield better restoration of function than later anastomosis or grafting, but this is only possible if the severed ends can be approximated without tension and if the wound is relatively uncontaminated.

Then, under stereomicroscopic visualization, careful fascicular alignment and two or three very fine nonabsorbable sutures through a nerve the size of the recurrent laryngeal or more such sutures through the epineurium of larger nerves may be successful. If primary anastomosis is not feasible, repair may be attempted in the subsequent few weeks, the permissible delay being a function of the length of the distal segment of the severed nerve and hence the duration and degree of muscle atrophy. If the proximal and distal segments of the nerve cannot be approximated without tension, even by mobilization to the extent possible, an autologous graft, or cross-grafting,[30] is the only recourse. Because the regenerating axons have to bridge two gaps in grafts versus only one in anastomosis, and because fascicular alignment is not possible, restoration of function will generally be less after grafting than after anastomosis.

Injuries to the parotid gland should be considered potential threats to the facial nerve. More than any other nerve this deserves repair by careful reapproximation with interrupted, fine, synthetic, nonabsorbable suture, using when necessary, autogenous nerve interposition grafting. Chances for success are better with this nerve and its loss of function is obvious and significantly consequential.[7]

Injury to the thyroid gland usually requires no more than that necessitating hemostasis and occasionally debridement.

Surely, the future will see nerve repair in gunshot wounds gaining greater consideration, especially for such critical innervations as that of the larynx and as the mechanisms of axoplasmic transport and axon regeneration become clearer.[31]

SUMMARY

The neck is a region relatively frequently and relatively seriously wounded by firearms. As in other regions of the body, wounds by firearms have, in American "civil" life, become more frequent than knife wounds and carry higher mortality. We believe, although there is controversy, that all penetrating gunshot wounds of the neck should be explored, since that site, particularly, yields a high incidence of false-positive and false-negative diagnoses preoperatively. Probing entrance and exit wounds, other than to identify penetration of the platysma muscle, is dangerous, uninformative, and a practice to be condemned.[1,9] Similarly to be condemned is blind clamping of vessels, since digital control is as effective and is atraumatic.[1] In the preoperative assessment of such injuries, radiographic examination of the neck must include both anterior-posterior and lateral views to identify metallic fragments and to evaluate possible cervical spine or spinal cord injury. As in other regions of the body, the cavities above and below the neck wound warrant similar radiographic evaluation. Concern for spinal cord injury takes precedence over all other concerns in neck wounds, assuming fatal exsanguination and asphyxiation are not imminent. Unless there is evidence of ischemic damage to the brain, common or internal carotid arterial injuries should be repaired. Conversely, internal jugular venous injuries can be treated by ligation. Salvageable injuries to the respiratory tract in the neck are relatively uncommon and are best managed by primary repair or conversion to a tracheostomy. Penetrating wounds of the esophagus are invariably fatal unless adequate drainage prevents mediastinitis. In the management of all of these injuries of the neck, entrance and exit wounds can be debrided and closed primarily.

REFERENCES

1. Saletta, J.D., Lowe, R.J., Lim, L.T. et al. Penetrating trauma of the neck. *J Trauma.* 16:579–587, 1976.
2. Knightly, J.J., Swaminathan, A.P., and Rush, B.F. Management of penetrating wounds of the neck. *Am J Surg.* 126:575–580, 1973.
3. Ashworth, C., Williams, L.F., and Byrne, J.J. Penetrating wounds of the neck: reemphasis of the need for prompt exploration. *Am J Surg.* 121:387–391, 1971.
4. Jones, R.F., Terrell, J.C., and Salyer, K.E. Penetrating wounds of the neck: an analysis of 274 cases. *J Trauma.* 7:228–237, 1967.
5. Sheely, C.H., Mattox, K.L., Reul, G.J. et al. Current concepts in the management of penetrating neck trauma. *J Trauma.* 15:895–900, 1975.
6. Blass, D.C., James, E.C., Reed, R.J. et al. Penetrating wounds of the neck and upper thorax. *J Trauma.* 18:2–7, 1978.
7. De la Cruz, A., and Chandler, J.R. Management of penetrating wounds of the neck. *Surg Gynecol Obstet.* 137:458–460, 1973.
8. Lau, J.M., Mattox, K.L., Beall, A.C. et al. Use of substitute conduits in traumatic vascular injury. *J Trauma.* 17:541–546, 1977.
9. Stein, A., and Kalk, F. Selective conservatism in the management of penetrating wounds of the neck. *Suid-Afrikaanse Tydskrif vir Chirurgie.* 12:31–40, 1974.
10. Bricker, D.L., Noon, G.P., Beall, A.C. et al. Vascular injuries of the thoracic outlet. *J Trauma.* 10:1–15, 1970.
11. Cohen, A., Brief, D., and Mathewson, C. Carotid artery injuries: an analysis of 85 cases. *Am J Surg.* 120:210–214, 1970.
12. Fitchett, V.H., Pomerantz, M., Butsch, D.W. et al. Penetrating wounds of the neck: a military and civilian experience. *Arch Surg.* 99:307–314, 1969.
13. Williams, J.W., and Sherman, R.T. Penetrating wounds of the neck: surgical management. *J Trauma.* 13:435–442, 1973.

14. Flax, R.L., Fletcher, H.S., and Joseph, W.L. The management of penetrating neck injuries. *Rev Surg.* 30:218-219, 1973.

15. *Emergency War Surgery. U.S. Armed Forces Issue of NATO Handbook.* Prepared for use by the Medical Services of NATO Nations. Washington, D.C.: U.S. Government Printing Office, 1958.

16. Maughon, J.S. An inquiry into the nature of wounds resulting in killed in action in Vietnam. *Milit Med.* 135:8-13, 1970.

17. Ducker, T.B., and Byrnes, D.P. Immediate mini-myelogram in acute cord injury. *J Trauma.* (In press). Presented at the 39th Annual Meeting of the American Association for the Surgery of Trauma. Chicago, September 13-15, 1979.

18. Levy, B.I., Valladares, W.R., Ghaem, A. et al. Comparison of plethysmographic methods with pulsed Döppler blood flowmetry. *Am J Physiol.* 236:H899-H903, 1979.

19. Hunt, T.K. Blaisdell, F.W., and Okimoto, J. Vascular injuries of the base of the neck. *Arch Surg.* 98:586-590, 1969.

20. Amato, J.J., Rich, N.M., Billy, L.J. et al. High velocity arterial injury: a study of the mechanism of injury. *J Trauma.* 11:412-416, 1971.

21. Shirkey, A.L., Beall, A.C., and DeBakey, M.E. Surgical management of penetrating wounds of the neck. *Arch Surg.* 86:955-963, 1963.

22. Stone, H.H., and Callahan, G.S. Soft tissue injuries of the neck. *Surg Gynecol Obstet.* 117:745-752, 1963.

23. Chiu, C.J., Terzis, J., and MacRae, M.L. Replacement of superior vena cava with the spiral composite vein graft. *Ann Thorac Surg.* 17:555-560, 1974.

24. Swan, K.G. (ed.). *Venous Surgery in the Lower Extremities.* St. Louis, Mo.: Warren H. Green Publishing Co., 1975.

25. Carter, R., Wareham, E.E., and Brewer, L.A. Rupture of the bronchus following closed chest trauma. *Am J Surg.* 104:177-195, 1962.

26. Urschel, H.C., and Razzuk, M.A. Management of acute traumatic injuries of tracheobronchial tree. Collective Reviews. *Surg Gynecol Obstet.* 136:113-117, 1973.

27. Clerf, L.H. Paralysis of the larynx of peripheral origin. *Acta Otolaryngol.* 43:108-112, 1953.

28. Mountcastle, V.B. *Medical Physiology,* 13th Ed. St. Louis, Mo.: C.V. Mosby Co., 1974.

29. Sunderland, S. *Nerves and Nerve Injuries,* 2nd Ed. Edinburgh: Churchill Livingstone, 1979.

30. Smith, J.W., and Gillen, F.J. Current techniques in peripheral nerve repair. Edited by R.W. Rand. In *Microneurosurgery,* 2nd Ed. St. Louis, Mo.: C.V. Mosby Co., 1978.

31. Wilson, D.L., and Stone, G.C. Axoplasmic transport of proteins. *Am Rev Biophys Bioengineer.* 8:27-45, 1979.

6 The Chest

As experience increased in the management of penetrating chest trauma, the number of thoracotomies progressively decreased.*

Trauma to the chest may be blunt or penetrating. It may surprise some that the reported experience reveals that blunt trauma is apparently more life-threatening than penetrating trauma.[1] Two reasons for this difference are: (1) blunt trauma is less obvious and diagnosis more likely to be in error; and (2) for blunt trauma to appear as a statistic, there must be significant dysfunction and injury. This distinction must be considered when comparing reports of results of chest trauma and its management. Since both types of trauma may occur simultaneously, principles and procedures appropriate to the diagnosis and management of each may have to be modified and compromised when the wound or wounds combine characteristics of both.

---

*Beall, A.C., Bricker, D.L., Crawford, H.W. et al. Considerations in the management of penetrating thoracic trauma. *J Trauma.* 8:408–417, 1968.

In recent years, gunshot wounds of the chest have become more frequent in United States civil life than all other forms of chest trauma. In a recent report of a large series of chest injuries,[2] 63% of penetrating wounds were caused by firearms. In a large series which included both blunt trauma and penetrating wounds of the chest, guns accounted for 59% of the injuries.[3]

Penetrating gunshot wounds to civilians in this country are much greater threats to survival than are knife wounds because they almost always involve penetration of the pleura, and because much more kinetic energy is usually dissipated.

In the Korean and Vietnam Wars, 35% and 37%, respectively, of fatal wounds were thoracic (Table 6-1). Only those of the head had higher mortality (41%). Somewhat surprising then, is the generally accepted statistic that only 15% of penetrating chest injuries require open thoracotomy. This figure is in marked contrast to that associated with penetrating gunshot wounds of the abdomen, almost all of which require laparotomy, as will be discussed in the next chapter. The chest is, in fact, the only region of the body which is not usually explored in the case of penetrating gunshot wounds. As we have already discussed, penetrating wounds of the head and neck are usually explored, as are penetrating gunshot wounds of the extremities. This high mortality rate from thoracic trauma and the infrequency of surgical intervention may seem paradoxical. An understanding of the relevant pathophysiology resolves this paradox.

Table 6-1
Anatomic Location of Fatal Wounds

	Korea[22] (%)	Vietnam[21] (%)
Head	41	39.3
Neck	5	7.3
Thorax	35	37.0
Abdomen	10	9.0
Upper Extremity	2	1.7
Lower Extremity	7	5.7

EMERGENCY DIAGNOSIS AND THERAPY

In addition to emergency concerns and procedures relevant to any serious injury (see Chapter 3), the most important consideration in a gunshot wound of the chest is the quality of breath sounds on auscultation of the chest. Decreased breath sounds suggest hemothorax, hemopneumothorax, or pneumothorax. The treatment is the same for each, and tube thoracostomy is justified on the basis of this clinical finding alone, particularly if vital signs are unstable. If vital signs are normal and stable, radiographic confirmation is appropriate. A physician must attend the patient through radiography, since the patient's condition may deteriorate rapidly. Optimally, posterior-anterior and lateral radiograms should be taken with the patient erect. However, the patient may not tolerate the erect position. One must remember that the convenience of a supine anterior-posterior radiogram is offset by its unreliability. As much as a liter of fluid in the pleural cavity initially may go unrecognized in this view. The dilemma is resolved by resort to a lateral decubitus radiogram with the injured side dependent. Thus, the two main indications for tube thoracostomy are auscultatory and radiographic.

It is often stated that aspiration of blood upon thoracentesis is also an indication. The indications for the procedure are those for tube thoracostomy; however, we do not think it is useful in the diagnosis or management of chest trauma. Thoracentesis, while it is diagnostic, will usually prove too slow for the volume of blood or the rate of internal bleeding. Thus, thoracentesis does not allow for sufficiently rapid pulmonary reexpansion to arrest hemorrhage from the collapsed lung. As such, it will contribute to exsanguination and be worse than no intervention at all. In addition, thoracentesis may induce pneumothorax through inadvertent injury to pulmonary parenchyma.

Oparah and Mandal make an important point in advocating primary closure of penetrating chest injuries, and one which we believe deserves emphasis.[4] "Sucking wounds of the chest" must be a rarity; they note that they have never seen one, despite considerable experience in the field. Nonetheless, the potential exists and can be best obviated by suture closure of the entrance wound. Even relatively high-velocity missile wounds tolerate this technique. As in wounds to the head, face, neck, and external genitalia, debridement and primary closure are empirically successful. Treatment of tangential high velocity gunshot wounds of the chest is based on principles which apply to other parts of the body: debridement and delayed primary closure (Figure 6-1–6-9).

A further point made by Oparah and Mandal relates to diaphragmatic injury; more precisely, injury to the left hemidiaphragm, with its threat of attendant herniation of abdominal contents into the left pleural space. Auscultation may fail to detect this pathologic problem because of the paralytic ileus which usually attends these injuries. However, a clue to the diagnosis is the appearance of peritoneal lavage fluid from the tube thoracostomy.

Tube thoracostomy is best performed with the patient supine and the upper extremity fully abducted. This position elevates the ribs and widens intercostal spaces. It also facilitates preparing a sterile field.

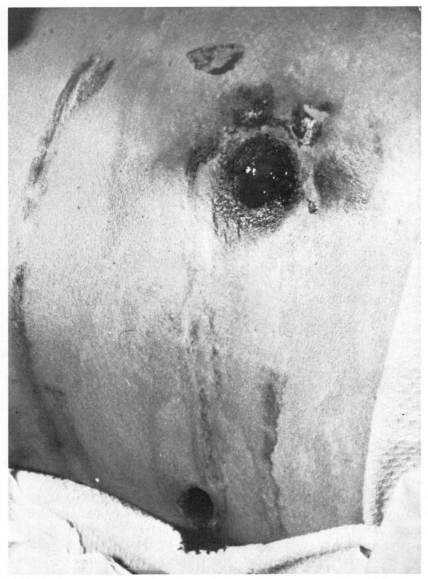

Figure 6-1 A 19-year-old soldier sustained an M-16 wound of the left chest from approximately 1 m away. The entrance wound (anterior and surrounded with powder burns) is larger than the exit wound (posterior).

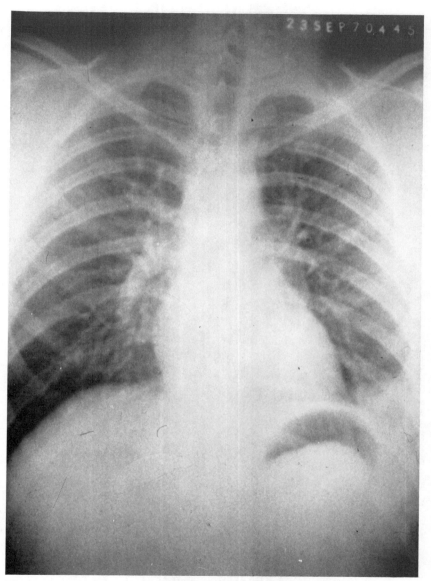

Figure 6-2 Chest radiogram reveals a left pleural effusion. Splenic injury was suspected clinically and was thought to be the cause of the effusion. A more probable explanation (and one indicating tube thoracostomy) was pulmonary parenchymal injury (contusion).

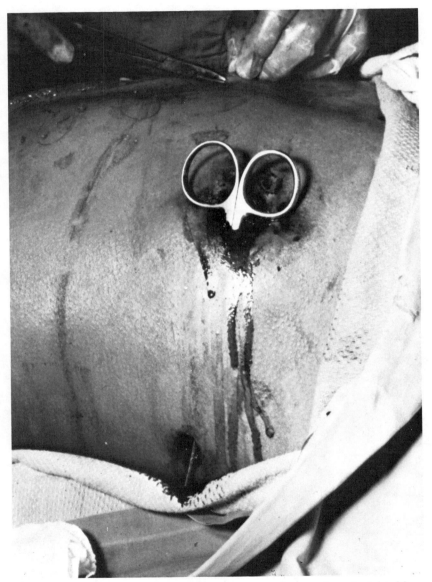

Figure 6-3 Exploratory laparotomy was negative, and a straight Mayo scissors (analogous to a bullet probe) has been passed through the bullet path and indicates the tangential nature of the chest wounds.

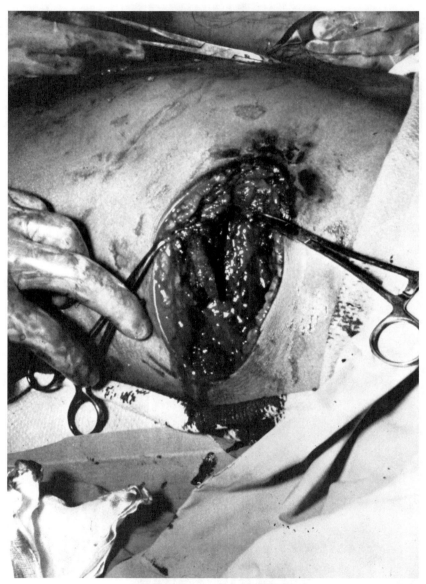

Figure 6-4   The skin overlying the wound tract is incised, and the underlying devitalized muscle is excised.

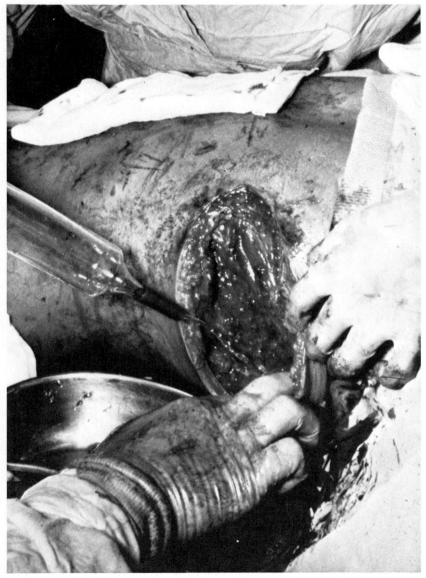

Figure 6-5 The debrided wound is injected with copious quantities of saline.

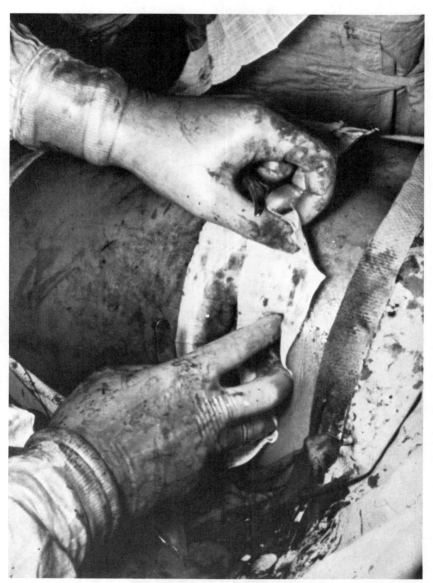

Figure 6-6   The wound is dressed with fine-mesh gauze to provide a relatively occlusive dressing while simultaneously permitting necessary wound drainage.

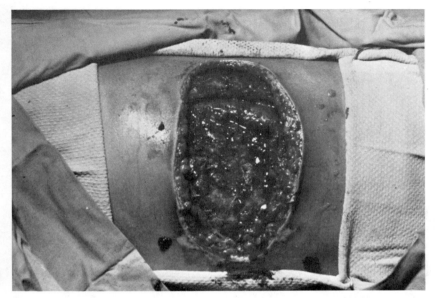

Figure 6-7   Five days later, the patient is returned to the operating room for delayed primary closure of this wound.

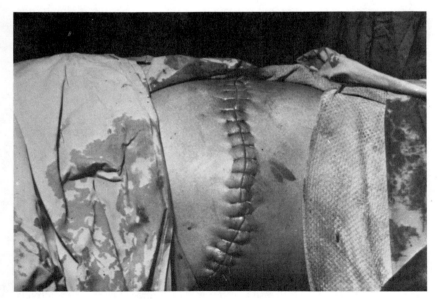

Figure 6-8   Closure is accomplished with through-and-through, fine stainless steel wire.

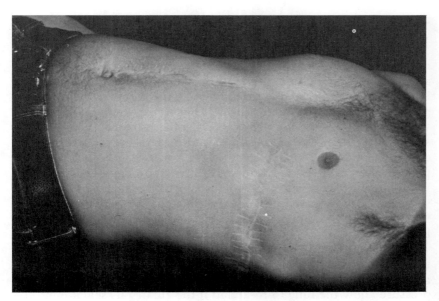

Figure 6-9 One year later, the patient is photographed to indicate a satisfactory cosmetic result to this relatively crude method of wound closure.

The chest tube is inserted more caudally and more posteriorly for suspected hemothorax than for pneumothorax, usually in the seventh intercostal space in the midaxillary line. At this level, there is no significant danger to the long thoracic nerve and relatively little to the liver or spleen. If the tube is inserted more posteriorly, the patient may turn on it and obstruct it.

The optimal site for insertion of the chest tube has been controversial. Most have advocated a posterior, dependent location when trauma indicates tube thoracostomy. Disagreement derives from knowledge that the pleural cavity is a closed space where pressure is below atmospheric during all phases of normal respiration. Thus, the intercostal space selected for insertion of the chest tube should not be important. To test this hypothesis, Hegarty[5] randomized into two groups patients who sustained penetrating chest trauma. One group was treated with tube thoracostomy via the second intercostal space in the midclavicular line; the other group, tube thoracostomy via the fifth intercostal space in the midaxillary line. There was no discernible difference in patient care, morbidity, or mortality, when chest tube position was the only variable.

If the patient is conscious, local anesthesia (1% lidocaine) will be required. A 1.5-inch, 22-gauge needle is better for injecting local anesthesia than a smaller needle, because of the thickness of the chest wall. Beyond this, the only instrument necessary is a #10 Bard-Parker scalpel blade. Blunt dissection using a curved clamp, is painful, unnecessary, and carries the risk of tearing the lung if pleural adhesions are present. The incision, optimally parallel to, and along the upper border of the lower rib, is carried down to the pleura and enlarged to permit entry of the index finger. Digital exploration determines whether the lung has retracted or whether there are local pleural adhesions. Blind insertion of the tube with a large curved clamp risks damage to the lung or heart and is painful. A #36 French, or comparable chest tube, is inserted to a depth of approximately six inches.

If hemothorax exists, there will usually be a gush of dark red blood through the thoracostomy. To the uninitiated, this may generate fear that he has created the intrathoracic hemorrhage. However, such hemorrhage is to be expected in a hemothorax attending gunshot wounds of the chest. Not uncommonly, as much as two liters of blood may quickly drain through the chest tube, following which drainage may abruptly stop. Drainage of this blood and release of intrapleural pressure allow the lung to reexpand if the cutaneous seal around the tube is complete. Thus, the tube should be sutured in place and attached to an underwater seal, suction, or Heimlich valve.[6]

The blood which drains from a chest tube inserted for penetrating trauma will usually be dark red for two reasons: (1) its source may be pulmonary arterial (relatively unoxygenated); and (2) alveolar exchange of oxygen in the collapsed lung is drastically reduced, and even pulmonary venous blood may be relatively unoxygenated. It has long been recognized empirically that a lacerated collapsed lung will usually continue to bleed, whereas, bleeding from the reexpanded lung usually stops abruptly. The mechanism of neither of these two phenomena is clearly understood. Continued bleeding from a collapsed, lacerated lung into a pleural cavity which has a volume of two to three liters plus the additional volume generated by mediastinal shift, can be rapidly exsanguinating, and can result from even minor pulmonary lacerations, if they go unattended.

If the blood draining from the chest tube is bright red, the source may be an intercostal artery, an internal thoracic artery, the aorta, or the left side of the heart. On the other hand, this blood may come from a laceration of the lung and may have been fully oxygenated by agitation within a hemopneumothorax. Such air contains oxygen at partial pressures approaching 144 mm Hg (0.20 [760–40] mm Hg). This is substantially higher than the oxygen tension in systemic arterial blood (80 to 100 mm Hg) (Tables 6-2, 6-3, and 6-4). When doubt exists regarding the source of blood drainage from a chest tube, analysis of the blood for the partial pressure of O_2 and CO_2 may provide a clue.[7]

Table 6-2
Partial Pressure of Oxygen (mm Hg)

Groups (Five dogs each)		Aorta	Pulmonary Artery	Chest Tube
I (Stab wound)	Control	89.4 ± 3.9 (S.E.)	37.4 ± 2.3	—
	Experimental	72.6 ± 4.2	40.6 ± 1.6	41.0 ± 1.2
II (Thoracotomy and lung laceration)	Control	90.2 ± 5.5	49.8 ± 4.3	—
	Experimental	71.0 ± 7.6*	40.6 ± 2.2*	146.0 ± 2.1*
III (Gunshot wound)	Control	91.2 ± 8.4	49.6 ± 5.5	—
	Experimental	84.4 ± 7.0	43.8 ± 6.4	48.8 ± 4.3
IV (Thoracotomy and pulmonary arterial blood injection)	Control	110.4 ± 3.3	59.0 ± 5.2	—
	Experimental	81.6 ± 4.8†	35.8 ± 2.2‡	82.1 ± 1.5†‡

Source: Swan, K.G. et al. Clinical implications of blood gas analysis on chest tube drainage. *J Trauma.* 19:823-827, 1979.
*Significantly different, p < 0.05
†Not significantly different, p > 0.05
‡Significantly different, p < 0.001

Table 6-3
Blood Gas Analyses of Patients Without Pneumothorax Treated for Penetrating Chest Trauma with Tube Thoracostomy

The data reveal a pO_2 of chest-tube drainage (blood) not significantly different from aortic blood pO_2.

	Aorta	Vena Cava	Chest Tube
pO_2	80.5*	28.9	61.7*
pCO_2	35.9	36.4	32.9
pH	7.36	7.35	7.30

Source: Swan, K.G. et al. Clinical implications of blood gas analysis on chest tube drainage. *J Trauma*. 19:823–827, 1979.
*Not significantly different, $p > 0.05$

Table 6-4
Analysis of a Similar Group of Patients with Pneumothorax Associated with Penetrating Chest Trauma

The data reveal a pO_2 of chest-tube blood which is significantly above that of aortic blood, indicating that the chest-tube drainage, color, and O_2 content may reflect the presence of concomitant pneumothorax, as well as possible systemic arterial or left-side-of-heart injury.

	Aorta	Vena Cava	Chest Tube
pO_2	77.8 *	37.8	116*
pCO_2	33.8	36.9	45.2
pH	7.41	7.36	7.39

Source: Swan, K.G. et al. *J Trauma*. 19:823–827, 1979.
*Significantly different, $p < 0.01$

After the initial gush of blood from the pleural cavity, attention must be directed to the flow over ensuing minutes and hours. If the continuing flow is greater than 100 to 200 ml per hour, surgical exploration becomes urgent, regardless of the color of the blood.

If the chest tube drainage is bright red, and if significant pneumothorax can be excluded, thoracotomy is indicated to control bleeding from systemic thoracic arteries, or from the left side of the heart. Anterolateral thoracotomy through the ipsilateral fifth intercostal space may be all the exposure that is necessary to ligate an injured internal thoracic or intercostal artery. A more formal posterolateral thoracotomy may be required to repair more extensive injury to the airway, lung, heart, or great vessel. Median sternotomy is an alternative approach to emergency thoracotomy. If abdominal exploration is necessary, a separate abdominal incision is required.[1,4,8-11]

AUTOTRANSFUSION

Autotransfusion is particularly applicable to the emergency management of a gunshot wound of the chest. Introduced over a century and a half ago,[12] enthusiasm for the technique has waxed and waned as techniques of blood typing, cross matching, collection, storage, and administration have developed. The first reported use of autotransfusion for a gunshot wound of the chest was in 1917, when Elmendorf[13] autotransfused 300 ml of blood aspirated from the chest of a German soldier during World War I. Presently, a variety of sophisticated techniques and devices are available for a spectrum of situations where autologous blood is preferable to homologous blood.[14] In the following discussion, we will consider the application of autotransfusion only to gunshot wounds of the chest.

The advantages are numerous and include the following: (1) the blood is readily available, cross-matched, and free from pyrogens; (2) febrile and allergic reactions are avoided; (3) there is no risk of hepatitis or isoimmunization from homologous antigens; and (4) its platelet count is often near normal (as opposed to banked blood),[14] since the blood is usually collected and infused rapidly. In addition, blood obtained from the pleural cavity shortly after a gunshot wound has near normal 2,3–diphosphoglycerate levels (as opposed to banked blood); thus, oxygen delivery to tissues is better preserved with autotransfused than banked blood, which is very low in this compound.[15] Presumably, red cell survival will be near normal following autotransfusion of blood obtained from a pleural cavity[16]; however, this has not been affirmed.[14]

An important consideration today is cost. Banked blood is charged to the patient at a rate which ranges from $25.00 to $50.00 per unit. Autotransfused blood can be delivered with the use of the most sophisticated equipment for as little as $8.00 to $12.00 per unit, and for considerably less using basic equipment to be described.[17]

The pleural cavity is an ideal source of blood for autotransfusion for a further reason. Usually, blood resulting from hemorrhage in chest trauma does not clot, since it is defibrinated by visceral and parietal pleura, as well as the mechanical actions of the heart, lung, and diaphragm.[16] When there is hemorrhage into a pleural cavity from an injury to heart or great vessels, there may be insufficient time for defibrination.[17] It must be remembered that such injury accounts for less than 15% of cases of penetrating chest trauma. Thus, theoretically, in more than 85% of cases, autotransfusion can be carried out safely without anticoagulation.

Current autotransfusion devices range from the recently popularized "Cell Saver," which separates out red cells, washes, and resuspends them prior to patient infusion,[18] down to the simple technique of chest tube bottle inversion.[17] The former, but not the latter, requires special technical assistance,[18] which limits its applicability to chest trauma.

The simplest technique for emergency resuscitation, such as would characterize a penetrating thoracic injury (Figure 6-10), is designed to eliminate not only the use of suction and pumping devices, but in so doing, the threat of air embolus. The apparatus does not require any external source of power, does not require technical support, operates on gravity collection and return principles, and incorporates a Dacron-wool filter (40-micra) to minimize contamination with particulate matter.

The blood is collected and anticoagulated in a prearranged, self-contained, sterile unit which incorporates a standard large-bore (#36 French) chest tube attached to a Heimlich valve. The latter is connected to a length of tubing of a caliber sufficient to facilitate rapid egress of blood flow from the chest tube into the collection bag. Thus, both rapid evacuation of the pleural cavity, as well as rapid reinfusion of the collected blood is facilitated. For obvious reasons, the catheter connecting the collection bag (now the administration set when inverted) is of comparably large bore and attached to a large-caliber venous line preferably inserted in the arm opposite the injured chest. A

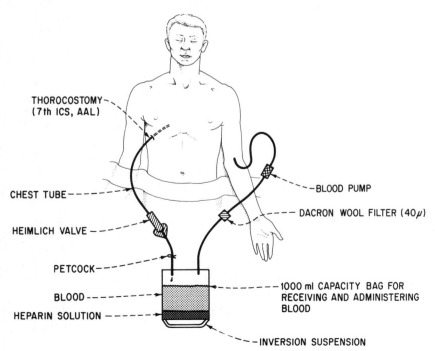

Figure 6-10 Autotransfusion device.

blood pump is an additional feature which will find useful application to the delivery line, since large volumes of blood administration are anticipated in such wounds. A pressure cuff can be applied to the administration set in the usual fashion to increase further the rate of infusion. Obviously, warming the blood is unnecessary with this technique. This method of autotransfusion is the simplest and safest of the techniques available. It is important to note that neither suction nor mechanical pump is needed. In contrast to techniques reported to date,[17,18] in the procedure described above, the force for evacuation of blood from the pleural cavity is provided by the patient's own respiratory movements.

The anticoagulant generally used is citrate-phosphate-dextrose solution (CPD),[19] at a ratio of one volume CPD to seven volumes of collected blood. Alternatively, acid-citrate-dextrose solution (ACD), or heparin may be used. We prefer heparin because it does not require refrigeration, whereas the other two solutions do. It remains to be demonstrated whether any anticoagulation is necessary. It is generally considered essential to add as an infusate, fresh frozen plasma and fresh platelets, if the volume of blood autotransfused is more than the patient's estimated normal circulating blood volume.[20] The low plasma fibrinogen concentration resulting from autotransfusion of blood obtained from the pleural cavity is not of serious concern, since the liver rapidly restores the deficit within hours to days.[14]

THORACOTOMY

Bright red or continued bleeding from the chest tube (Figures 6-11–6-24); persistent or uncontrolled air leak through the tube; apparent injury to the esophagus, tracheobronchial tree, heart, or great vessels; and persistence of significant amounts of blood in the pleural cavity[8,9] are all indications for thoracotomy. This is preferably performed in the operating room, but may have to be initiated in the emergency room.

The need for thoracotomy in the management of chest trauma is surprisingly infrequent; the response to tube thoracostomy is surprisingly good. In a large civilian series of such patients, Beall and associates[8,9] resorted to thoracotomy in only 5% of cases. When the need for late thoracotomy was included, the incidence rose to only 17%. The majority in this patient series sustained stab wounds, the remainder gunshot wounds. Respective mortality rates were 3% and 14%. When civilian chest trauma was restricted to penetrating gunshot wounds, in another large series, Borja and Ransdell[11] reported a thoracotomy rate of 19% and a mortality rate of 14%.

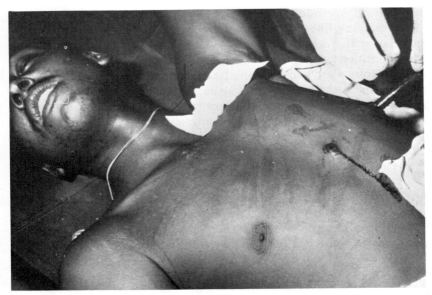

Figure 6-11 A 20-year-old soldier sustained a 45-caliber pistol wound of the chest from a distance of 1 m. Left tube thoracostomy was indicated by decreased left breath sounds on comparative auscultation of right and left chests.

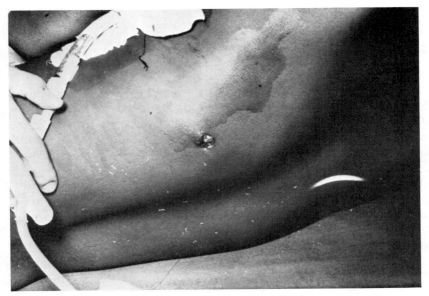

Figure 6-12 The exit wound is seen in the left back.

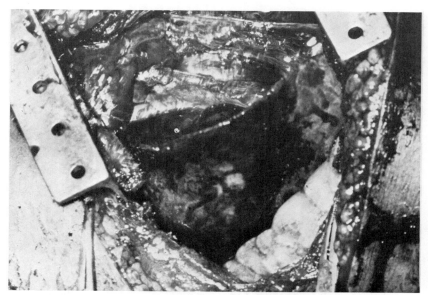

Figure 6-13 Because of suspected significant intrathoracic injury (based upon continued left chest-tube drainage of dark blood), the left chest was explored via an anterolateral thoracotomy through the fifth intercostal space. The left lower lobe of the lung is contused and cyanotic. The upper lobe is normal in appearance.

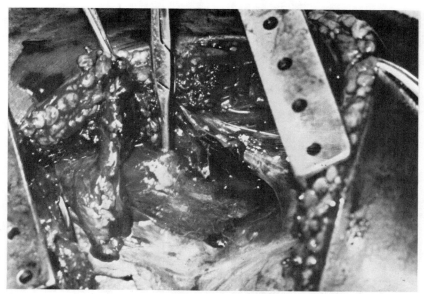

Figure 6-14 A defect in the pericardium is identified with the tip of the Mayo scissors.

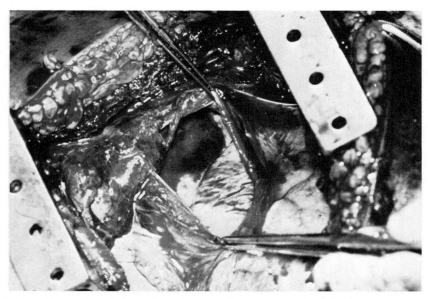

Figure 6-15 The pericardium is opened anterior to the left phrenic nerve, and a contusion of the diaphragmatic portion of the pericardium is observed and proved to be associated with a defect in the left hemidiaphragm. The heart was not injured.

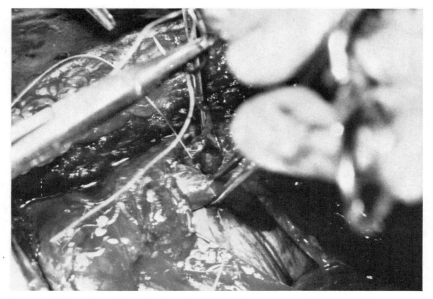

Figure 6-16 The defect in the diaphragm is closed with heavy (#0), nonabsorbable suture and mandates exploratory laparotomy.

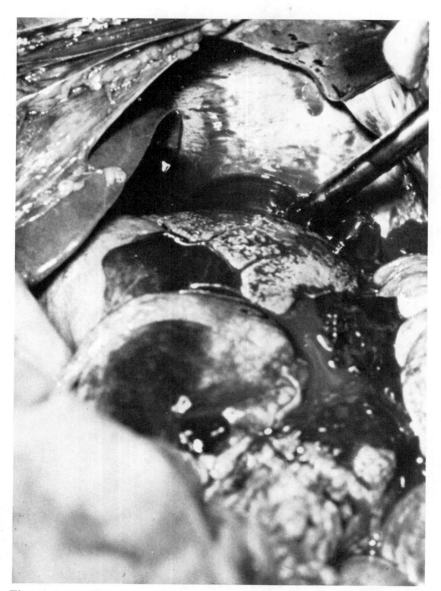

Figure 6-17 The abdomen has been explored and an injury to the spleen observed. The sucker tip points to a large blood clot on the lateral aspect of the spleen.

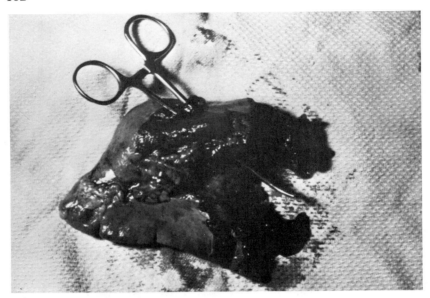

Figure 6-18 The spleen is removed, and the curved clamp identifies the path of the bullet.

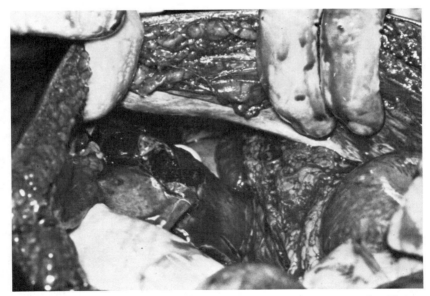

Figure 6-19 An associated injury to the left lobe of the liver is identifed.

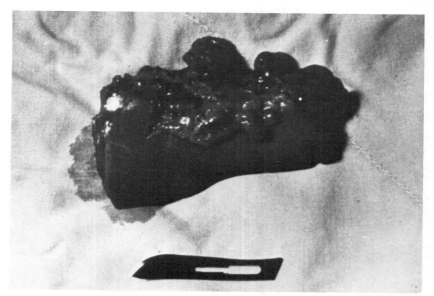

Figure 6-20 Left hepatic lobectomy is carried out, and the specimen is exhibited alongside a #10 Bard-Parker scalpel blade for size comparison.

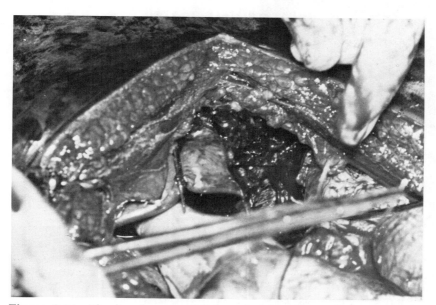

Figure 6-21 Bleeding from the left hepatic lobe is controlled with suture ligatures of 0-chromic catgut.

104

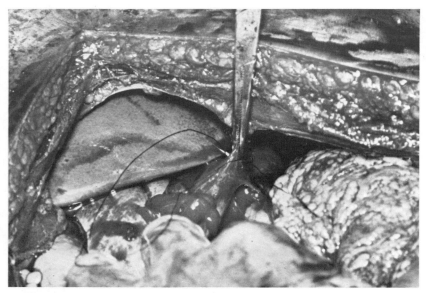

Figure 6-22 An associated small hole in the stomach is closed with interrupted 3-0 silk.

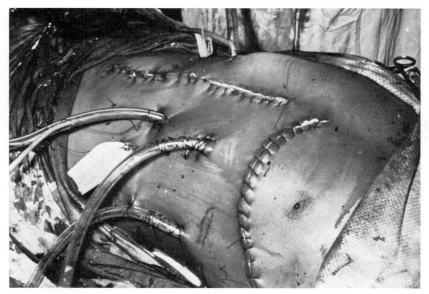

Figure 6-23 The wounds have all been closed; two chest tubes are in place. Sump tubes drain the splenic bed and left hepatic lobe region along with multiple Penrose drains which allow for relatively early removal (after 48 to 72 hours) of the sump tubes. Sump tubes are a threat to hollow viscera and may cause perforation if left in place too long.

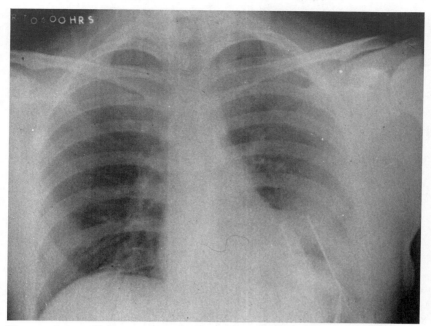

Figure 6-24 Chest radiogram performed after surgery reveals a left pulmonary contusion and presence of the two chest tubes. In this case, thoracotomy was unnecessary.

Blunt trauma to the chest generally increases the need for thoracotomy and the mortality of any series of chest wounds. Nonetheless, Kish and associates,[1] in another large series of patients with chest trauma, reported an initial thoracotomy rate of 12% and a late thoracotomy rate of an additional 4%. The overall mortality was 3%. In analyzing a series of such patients in the Vietnam War, McNamara[10] reported an initial thoracotomy rate of 11% to 12% and an ultimate thoracotomy rate of 14% to 16%. The attendant mortality rates were 1.7% to 4.3%. If thoracotomy is used more aggressively in the management of penetrating chest trauma, as some advocate, results are not improved.

In reviewing our experience in an urban ghetto with penetrating thoracic trauma secondary to gunshot and knife wounds, but specifically excluding blunt trauma, we found an overall thoracotomy rate of 35%, more than twice what we would recommend based upon the published experience (Table 6-5). In our series, there were 100 stab wounds and 50 gunshot wounds. Patients with stab wounds fared better; nevertheless, the overall mortality for the series exceeded 17%, and even more important, thoracotomy, whether implemented to manage stab wounds or gunshot wounds (Table 6-5), was associated with a sizable mortality rate. If a fatality occurred, there was an 80%

chance that thoracotomy preceded it; similarly, if a thoracotomy was. performed in the patient's management, the chance of a fatal outcome was 47%. The figures serve to emphasize the judicious use of chest exploration in management of penetrating thoracic trauma.

Next to the head the chest is the most vulnerable target in combat.[21,22] Because of their size, the lungs are the most frequently injured viscera in gunshot wounds of the chest. As mentioned, most such pulmonary injuries respond to tube thoracostomy alone.

Table 6-5
A More Aggressive Approach to Penetrating Chest Injuries (Those Requiring Tube Thoracostomy)
The data reveal an overall mortality of 17%, compared to a thoracotomy rate of 35%, which was associated with a mortality rate of 46%. Coincidental exploratory laparotomy was required in 28% of these penetrating chest injuries.

	Mortality* (%)	Thoracotomy† (%)	Laparotomy‡ (%)
Knife	8	30	20
Gun	35	45	45
X̄ (Mean)	17	35	28

Source: Report of the Medical Audit Committee, College of Medicine and Dentistry of New Jersey, Harrison S. Martland Hospital, 1976.
*Thoracotomy—82%
†Mortality—46%
‡Mortality without thoracotomy—17%

LUNG

In World War I, it was recognized that excision of contused regions of the lungs reduced the incidence of lung abscess and empyema, complicating gunshot wounds of lungs.[23] In World War II, it was recognized that a large percentage of such cases of pulmonary contusion (see Figure 6-13) responded adequately to tube thoracostomy alone, and that the risks of emergency pulmonary resection exceeded the risks of abscess, empyema, or as eventually generally recognized in the Vietnam War, the "wet lung syndrome" ("posttraumatic pulmonary insufficiency," "shock lung" syndromes). In the Korean War, and subsequently in the Vietnam War, it became more generally recognized that despite the low density and higher extensibility of pulmonary parenchyma (conditions unfavorable to the dissipation of the kinetic energy of the missile) the concomitant pulmonary vascular damage somehow induced localized pulmonary parenchymal edema.[24-26]

Metabolic gas (O_2, CO_2) exchange across the thickness of the blood-gas barrier between alveoli and alveolar capillaries is inversely proportional to the thickness of the barrier (i.e., the diffusion distance).

Thus, the slightest degree of interstitial edema in this blood-gas barrier will dramatically curtail such gaseous exchange. Such edema may develop locally in regions of pulmonary contusion, as it does in other contused tissue. The resultant local hypoxia reflexly induces a shunting of pulmonary arterial blood from such contused regions to initially undamaged regions of the lungs. Eventually, however, through mechanisms not understood, together with the effects of over-energetic administration of blood or physiologic solution, interstitial edema develops in uninjured regions of the lung and produces severe hypoxemia. It follows, then, that restitution of plasma volume is best accomplished by colloid-containing solutions rather than by isotonic crystalloid solutions. However, experience has not confirmed this deduction.* From an analysis of cases of penetrating thoracic injuries in the Vietnam War, Fischer recommended resection of the contused pulmonary tissue if the systemic arterial pO_2 could not be maintained above 40 mm Hg, despite "vigorous pulmonary supportive measures" including endotracheal O_2 in high concentration.[24]†

When pulmonary parenchymal injury results from gunshot and thoracotomy is indicated, suture plication of the wound would seem indicated; but, this procedure is rarely satisfactory. It is difficult to control bleeding or air leak with this technique. This observation further supports the convictions that pulmonary parenchymal injury usually responds to tube thoracostomy alone, and that there are obvious disadvantages to thoracotomy for control of such injuries. Blood loss alone is an important consideration. Since collapse of a lacerated lung aggravates bleeding, thoracotomy can be expected to encourage bleeding from pulmonary parenchymal injury. We believe that if treatment of comparable pulmonary parenchymal gunshot wounds is divided into those managed by tube thoracostomy and those managed by thoracotomy and suture ligation, the blood lost in the former group will be significantly less than that in the latter group. We estimate this ratio, as measured by blood replacement, will approximate 2:3. To our knowledge, this hypothesis has not been tested.

When pulmonary parenchymal injury is extensive, resection of a lobe or an entire lung may be required. Whether this more aggressive approach will reduce or eliminate the complication of late abscess formation and the need for delayed pulmonary resection, is not clear from available information to date.

---

*Virgilio, R.W., Rice, C.L., Smith, D.E. et al. Crystalloid vs colloid resuscitation: is one better? *Surgery* 85:129–139, 1979.
†Fischer and associates compared results of nonoperative and pulmonary resectional therapy for pulmonary contusion due to penetrating missiles. They observed a 100% mortality in the unoperated patients vs a 12% mortality in the surgical group. Although the authors concluded that because of the small sample size this difference was not statistically significant, in fact the difference *is highly significant* ($p < 0.001$, Fischer's exact test).

When tube thoracostomy fails to drain blood adequately from the pleural cavity, thoracotomy is indicated to prevent empyema and/or resultant fibrous encapsulation of the lung.[8]

Empyema continues to complicate chest trauma, regardless of the precise mode of therapy. Consideration of empyema is reintroduced at this time to provide some guidelines, not to its prophylaxis, which has been discussed, but rather to its management. This can be quite vexing, mainly because of indecision as to when to operate. In a large series of patients with chest trauma, Arom et al have distinguished the empyema that accompanies a simple clotted hemothorax, such as might accompany an inadequately drained penetrating chest injury, and that which they call an infected organizing hemothorax.[27] Admittedly, the distinction is relatively subtle, but the management is critical. Six percent of this series of 300 patients developed post-traumatic empyema. Fifteen percent of the 300 patients developed clotted hemothorax. The authors make the important point that the so-called "peel," or fibrous entrapment of the lung within the pleural space and subsequent to the empyema, develops within one to three weeks. At this time, the lesion is amenable to excision, allowing full expansion of the lung. If excision is delayed until six weeks, a tough, organized, fibrous layer replaces this peel, and a much more formidable decortication is required to accomplish the same goal.

The above principles of management of gunshot wounds of the lung (prompt and appropriate resort to tube thoracostomy, thoracotomy when evidence of retained blood or blood clot follows tube thoracostomy, resection of contused pulmonary parenchyma in the face of severe hypoxemia, and possibly prophylactic antibiotics) should reduce the incidence of late complications of gunshot wounds of the lungs, such as fibrous encapsulation and the need for ultimate surgical decortication.

TRACHEOBRONCHIAL TREE

Penetrating injury to the tracheobronchial tree, whether due to gunshot, fragment, or knife, constitutes a serious threat to pulmonary function. Such an injury is heralded by: (1) subcutaneous emphysema; (2) cough; (3) hemoptysis; (4) pneumothorax; (5) dyspnea; (6) xyphisternal crunch (Hamman sign) on auscultation; (7) massive air leak following tube thoracostomy; (8) progressive or uncontrolled air leak (a cardinal sign of tracheal or bronchial rupture).[28] Failure to identify such injuries and to repair them at the time of the initial injury results in delayed sequellae such as bronchial or tracheal stenosis and ultimate loss of associated pulmonary function secondary to lobar collapse, atelectasis, and atresia. If the patient survives the initial injury without surgical intervention, symptoms of respiratory distress usually follow within seven to ten days, as ingrowth of granulation tissue tends to seal the defect in the airway. At this point, tracheobronchial reconstruction becomes more formidable and may require lengthening procedures such as: (1) laryngeal release; (2) tracheal mobilization; (3) pulmonary hilar mobilization; and (4) division of the inferior pulmonary ligaments.[28]

Many cases of complete severance of a primary or secondary bronchus have not only been compatible with life, but have proven amenable to successful reconstruction two months to 15 years following initial injury.[29-31] A completely severed bronchus is sufficiently supported by surrounding parenchyma that it can adequately conduct air, provided hemorrhage does not interfere. A completely severed bronchus is better tolerated than a partially severed bronchus. When severance is complete, the pulmonary parenchyma which the former ventilates collapses. The lung becomes atelectatic and infection does not occur.[28] The blood supply to this pulmonary tissue is sufficient, despite the severed bronchus. Conversely, when partial tear of a bronchus occurs, the pulmonary tissue it aerates becomes infected and loss of parenchyma is likely.[28] Clearly, the earlier the attempt at repair of such injuries, the greater the likelihood of success. Thus, early use of bronchoscopy is advocated in the initial evaluation and ultimate management of potential tracheobronchial injuries.

The principles of management of injuries to the airway are described in Chapter 5. Injuries to the airway within the thorax are much more threatening. As with other penetrating injuries to the thorax, gunshot wounds of the tracheobronchial tree are associated with a much higher morbidity and mortality because damage and required debridement are more extensive, and because techniques available for replacement of the tracheobronchial defect are often inadequate.[32]

Tracheobronchial wounds, whether in the chest or the neck, can be repaired by fine nonabsorbable suture placed in interrupted fashion. Autosuturing techniques are also applicable. After the thoracic lesion is repaired, cervical tracheostomy is recommended to reduce inspiratory and expiratory resistance and to reduce pressure gradients across the suture line.

PROPHYLACTIC ANTIBIOTICS

The evidence accumulated over the past 40 years fails to demonstrate a decisive benefit from prophylactic antibiotics in gunshot wounds of the lungs.[33-36] Nevertheless, it is admittedly difficult to refrain from using them in penetrating wounds of the chest. If the decision is to use an antibiotic prophylactically, a broad-spectrum antibiotic, or combination of antibiotics, should be considered. A recent report[35] suggests some reduction in empyema when use or not of antibiotics is the variable following tube thoracostomy for penetrating injuries of the chest, but the differences are very small.

HEART

In past decades, stab wounds have been the most common form of penetrating trauma to the chest resulting in cardiac injury.[37,38] A more recent report indicates differently, that is, gunshot wounds are a more common cause of penetrating chest wounds leading to cardiac trauma.[39] A gunshot wound of the heart is more often fatal than is a stab wound to that organ.[39,40] In all probability, most patients with cardiac wounds, especially cardiac gunshot wounds, do not receive medical attention antemortem. This probability thus favors outcome of management among those who do arrive alive at a treatment facility. By definition, these patients have a cardiac injury which is least compatible with life. Their survival depends upon prompt recognition of the probable lesion and immediate institution of appropriate therapy. A successful outcome following management of such wounds is probably the most gratifying experience for the trauma team.

Prompt recognition of the cardiac wound is critical. Symptoms and signs include Beck's triad. This classic description associates the history of chest trauma with (1) distant heart sounds upon auscultation over the precordium; (2) evidence of systemic venous hypertension, such as distended neck veins; and (3) systemic arterial hypotension. Current information indicates not only that the last (systemic arterial hypotension) is a late and ominous finding, but that the presence of the triad in instances of tamponade is variable (35% to 65%).[39,41-44] Neither the presence or absence of pulsus paradoxus, nor electrocardiographic changes are reliable in diagnosing pericardial tamponade.[37-39] Once suspicion of either cardiac wound or pericardial tamponade arises, a decision as to remedial or definitive therapy must be acted upon immediately. The question posed is whether to resort to pericardiocentesis, pericardial window, or thoracotomy. This decision is derived from historic perspectives as well as current experience.

The German surgeon Rehn is generally given credit for the first successful repair of a cardiac wound.[45] The year was 1897, and the injury was a stab wound of the right ventricle. A wave of enthusiasm for operative management of all suspected heart wounds followed, but success was moderate (about 50% recovery)[45] and was related to stab, as opposed to gunshot, wounds. These results, coupled with studies in dogs which dated back to the time of Napoleon's surgeon, Larrey,[46] focused attention on the pathophysiology of pericardial tamponade and led to an alternative consideration in management, namely, pericardial aspiration or pericardiocentesis. Dogs, for example, were shown to sustain cardiovascular collapse associated with instilling 150 ml of saline in their pericardial cavities and yet they recovered following removal of as little as 20 ml of the same fluid.[47] Popularized in this country by Blalock and Ravitch[48] and others,[49] this form of therapy gained rapid acceptance and persisted as the procedure of choice until the mid-1960s. At about that time, traumatologists in both Dallas[40] and Houston[50] arrived at the conclusion that salvage rates could be even further improved if surgery was expeditiously carried out, often in the emergency room.[51] Maynard[52] had reached the same conclusion considerably earlier (1952).

Currently, a reasonable approach to wounds of the heart includes a combination of these techniques. If hemorrhagic hypotension from cardiac wounds is ruled out, and if pericardial tamponade is suspected, either pericardiocentesis,[38] or pericardial window[37] (each through a subxiphoid approach) is indicated. However, these two procedures should be performed only if time permits and as a preoperative adjunct to thoracotomy.

What is the nature of such wounds, how have the patients who sustained them fared, and what is the currently recommended therapy?

The right ventricle is most commonly the site of penetrating cardiac injury. Left ventricle, right atrium, and left atrium follow in order of frequency.[37-40] Injuries to the left ventricle carry the worst prognosis[40] in patients with suspected traumatic tamponade. Gunshot wounds are less likely to produce pericardial tamponade than are stab wounds because the former are more often associated with through-and-through injuries to both myocardium and pericardium.[43,44] This type of wound permits drainage of pericardial blood into a pleural cavity and stalls the development of tamponade. Pericardiocentesis is often associated with a significant incidence of false negative findings because pericardial blood often clots.[37,39,43,44,51] Since hemopericardium may progress to fibrous adhesions and chronic constrictive pericarditis, early evacuation by needle aspiration or pericardiostomy becomes critical. This complication is an additional justification for thoracotomy when pericardial tamponade is suspected.

A relatively subtle but potentially lethal injury to the heart is a tangential wound which produces little or no tamponade initially, but which does result in delayed rupture of the myocardium, acute tamponade, and death.[53,54] These possibilities further justify prompt surgical exploration for suspected wounds of the heart.

Cardiac arrest associated with penetrating chest injury is an additional indication for thoracotomy, often in the emergency room. The condition implies pericardial tamponade.[55] Speculation exists regarding the precise cause of cardiac arrest and sudden death attending penetrating chest injuries complicated by pericardial tamponade. Yao and associates,[56] as well as others,[42] proposed a reduction in right ventricular filling as the primary etiologic factor.

Once surgical intervention is decided upon, the question often arises as to the optimal surgical incision. We favor a left anterolateral thoracotomy through the fourth or fifth intercostal space (see Figure 6-11). This incision can be easily and expeditiously extended across to the right chest if necessary. The left thoracotomy provides for adequate exposure of pericardium and heart. The left hilum is also easily exposed for cross-clamping if exsanguinating pulmonary injury or massive air leak indicates this step. Similarly, the descending aorta can be readily cross-clamped through this incision. Descending aortic cross-clamping is also a valuable technique for assisting control of intraabdominal hemorrhage. Of even greater importance, it sustains cardiac output distribution to brain and myocardium when hypovolemic shock is developing.[57]

Nearly a century ago, Theodor Billroth admonished that ''a surgeon who tries to suture a heart wound deserves to lose the esteem of his colleagues.''[57] Almost a hundred years later, the trauma surgeon approaches such injury with trepidation. He knows that he will not be criticized for ''emergency room thoracotomy'' in the management of a gunshot wound of the chest. Nonetheless, he is cognizant of the fact that salvage rates today for wounds of the heart under such circumstances are relatively meager (8% to 24%).[57,58] Presumably, improvement is inevitable, but the question remains how? Eighty-one percent of homicides in this country are by gunshot and the heart is the most vulnerable target.[59]

ESOPHAGUS

Gunshot wounds of the thoracic esophagus are rarely encountered by the traumatologist because of the proximity of the esophagus to the aorta. Injury to the one is usually associated with injury to the other. A gunshot wound of the thoracic aorta will usually cause rapid and fatal exsanguination into one or both pleural cavities. Rapid asphyxiation occurs simultaneously. Despite its infrequency, injury to the thoracic esophagus must be diligently sought whenever a gunshot wound to the chest is treated. Several clues to the diagnosis assist the trauma surgeon.

Unilateral pleural effusion may be evident clinically as well as radiographically, and indicates probable escape of gastric contents refluxing up and through the esophageal tear. Pneumomediastinum may be evident clinically and radiographically, but is relatively rare. The nasogastric tube may be seen radiographically to extend into a pleural space instead of into the stomach. If a metallic fragment is seen in the posterior mediastinum radiographically, esophagography is indicated.[11] Water-soluble radiopaque contrast material instilled through the nasogastric tube just distal to the pharynx may appear in a pleural cavity. For obvious reasons, a barium swallow, although diagnostic, would be contraindicated. Methylene blue instilled in the proximal esophagus may appear in the drainage of a tube thoracostomy, once bleeding has stopped and the drainage becomes clear. Esophagoscopy may reveal the presence of blood or the actual injury, but is not essential for diagnosis and may inflict more damage.

Once the diagnosis is established, thoracotomy is indicated and the esophagus is then repaired. The technique of repair is not as critical an issue as the recognition of the injury and its drainage with tube thoracostomy. Failure to recognize a thoracoesophageal penetrating injury will result in empyema and usually death. Gastrostomy is indicated to prevent reflux of gastric contents into the esophagus and into the pleural cavity, since suture line dehiscence is common. Esophageal stricture is common following esophageal injury. Awareness of this fact has led some to advocate distal esophageal ligation at the time of thoracotomy and in place of gastrostomy to prevent gastric juice from entering the chest. We favor gastrostomy since it is usually adequate and esophageal ligation is permanent. The latter requires major surgical reconstruction to restore the alimentary tract. Cervical esophagostomy is required for salivary drainage if the distal esophagus is ligated; it will close spontaneously once distal obstruction is eliminated. Should thoracic esophageal stricture occur subsequent to injury and repair, dilation may be all that is required; however, formal resection and repair of the stricture may ultimately be necessary. Esophagogastrostomy, gastric tube, colon or small bowel interposition are all acceptable techniques of repair if resection of the stricture and primary anastomosis are not possible.

DIAPHRAGM

Approximately one in four penetrating chest injuries results in damage to the respiratory diaphragm.[9] For this reason, herniation into the pleural cavity of intraabdominal organs should be considered in the management of a gunshot or other wound of the chest. The left hemidiaphragm is most commonly involved.[60] The relatively large size of the liver and its coronary ligamentous attachments to the right hemidiaphragm limit herniation of the liver into the right pleural cavity. Also, the liver tends to obstruct or seal a defect in the diaphragm, thus preventing herniation of other abdominal organs into the right pleural space. Despite these factors limiting herniation on the right, its occurrence has been reported. On the other hand, a defect in the left hemidiaphragm may permit herniation of spleen, stomach, transverse colon, omentum, and even small bowel into the left pleural cavity. This syndrome can be detected on physical examination by auscultation of bowel sounds in the chest. The latter sign is uncommon because ileus resulting from the trauma usually silences the intestine.[4] Thus, absence of bowel sounds over the chest does not rule out such herniation.

P-A radiograms of the chest may reveal what appears to be an abnormally elevated diaphragm. Actually, the position of the dome of the diaphragm is not abnormal. The fundus of the gas-filled stomach is mistaken for diaphragm. A diagnosis of diaphragmatic paralysis secondary to phrenic nerve injury is entertained. Fluoroscopy may help resolve the confusion. The degree of herniation will appear to increase with inspiration. The importance of the nasogastric tube again becomes critical, since it can be seen radiographically and usually can be passed into the stomach, despite the herniation. Chest radiogram following injection of water-soluble radiographic contrast material such as sodium diatrizoate (Hypaque) through the nasogastric tube will identify the relationship of stomach and diaphragm. Instillation of air into the stomach via the nasogastric tube may be auscultated over the chest. If injury to the diaphragm is suspected, tube thoracostomy is indicated on the involved side. The injury may be confirmed by digital exploration at the time of thoracostomy, or identification of abdominal organs in the pleural space. The appearance of peritoneal lavage fluid from the chest tube is diagnostic of diaphragmatic penetration.[4] If herniation has occurred, laparotomy is mandatory.

Some have described reduction of the hernia and repair of the diaphragm during thoracotomy *without laparotomy*. We condemn this practice. As previously stated, a gunshot wound of the chest that penetrates the diaphragm demands exploratory laparotomy (see Figures 6-11–6-24). If herniation through the diaphragmatic injury is added, then the indication for abdominal exploration becomes even more imperative. Strangulation is likely. Thus, perforation of the intestine may be caused by either ischemia or the missile. Whether repaired from thoracic or abdominal sides, the injury to the diaphragm must be treated with heavy nonabsorbable suture such as #0 silk (see Figure 6-16). Interrupted mattress sutures closely spaced are recommended. The reason for this technique relates to reports of suture line disruption associated with diaphragmatic closure using simpler techniques and lighter or absorbable suture material. Despite its thinness, the respiratory diaphragm is a powerful muscle and a paroxysm of coughing or hiccoughing will severely stress any suture line in it.

SUMMARY

1. Gunshot wounds of the chest are now the most common injuries to that region.
2. Finding a relative decrease in breath sounds following a gun-

shot wound of the chest is an indication for tube thoracostomy on the same side.

3. Eighty-five percent of penetrating injuries to the chest respond to tube thoracostomy alone.

4. Rapid reexpansion of the injured lung is imperative, since the collapsed lung continues to bleed and fatal hemorrhage into a pleural cavity may result.

5. Tube thoracostomy drainage is usually dark red because it is relatively hypoxemic. This phenomenon results from collapse of the lung and the probable pulmonary arterial source of bleeding.

6. The converse, that is, drainage of bright red blood from a chest tube inserted for treatment of gunshot wound, should alert the physician to an alternative source of bleeding such as an injured thoracic systemic artery or left side of heart. These injuries require thoracotomy and surgical repair. An exception to this rule is significant pneumothorax which may allow systemic venous blood (dark red) to equilibrate with atmospheric air and become hyperoxemic (bright red).

7. Further indications for thoracotomy include cardiac arrest, suspected pericardial tamponade, suspected injury to heart or great vessel, uncontrolled air leak, persistent chest tube drainage of blood, esophageal injury, and failure of tube thoracostomy to evacuate all blood.

8. Diaphragmatic injury mandates exploratory laparotomy and closure with heavy nonabsorbable suture material.

9. Injuries to the thoracic esophagus require primary repair, tube thoracostomy, and gastrostomy.

REFERENCES

1. Kish, G., Kozloff, L., Joseph, W.L., et al. Indications for early thoracotomy in the management of chest trauma. *Ann Thorac Surg.* 22:23–28, 1976.

2. Robicsek, F., Sabbagh, A., Mullen, D.C., et al. Immediate surgery in the management of penetrating chest injuries. *J Cardiovasc Surg.* 13:156–159, 1972.

3. Reul, G.J., Mattox, K.L., Beall, A.C. et al. Recent advances in the operative management of massive chest trauma. *Ann Thorac Surg.* 16:52–66, 1973.

4. Oparah, S.S., and Mandal, A.K. Penetrating stab wounds of the chest: experience with 200 consecutive cases. *J Trauma.* 16:868–872, 1976.

5. Hegarty, M.M. A conservative approach to penetrating injuries of the chest: experience with 131 successive cases. *Injury.* 8:53–59, 1976.

6. Heimlich, H.J. Valve drainage of the pleural cavity. *Dis Chest.* 53:282–287, 1968.

7. Jain, K.M., Hastings, O.M., Saad, S.A. et al. Clinical implications of blood gas analysis of chest tube drainage. *J Trauma.* 19:823–827, 1979.

8. Beall, A.C., Bricker, D.L., Crawford, H.W. et al. Surgical management of penetrating thoracic trauma. *Dis Chest.* 49:568–577, 1966.

9. Beall, A.C., Bricker, D.L., Crawford, H.W. et al. Considerations in the management of penetrating thoracic trauma. *J Trauma.* 8:408–417, 1968.

10. McNamara, J.J., Messersmith, J.K., Dunn, R.A. et al. Thoracic injuries in combat casualties in Vietnam. *Ann Thorac Surg.* 10:389–401, 1970.

11. Borja, A.R., and Ransdell, H.T. Treatment of penetrating gunshot wounds of the chest: experience with 145 cases. *Am J Surg.* 122:81–84, 1971.

12. Blundell, J. Experiments on the transfusion of blood by the syringe. *Medico Chir Trans.* 9:56–92, 1818.

13. Elmendorf, D. Ueber wiederinfusion nach punktion eines frischen hämatothorax. *Munch Med Wochenschr.* 64:36–37, 1971.

14. Bell, W. The hematology of autotransfusion. *Surgery* 84:695–699, 1978.

15. Orr, M. Autotransfusion: the use of washed red cells as an adjunct component therapy. *Surgery* 84:728–730, 1978.

16. Symbas, P.N. Autotransfusion from hemothorax: experimental and clinical studies. *J Trauma.* 12:689–695, 1972.

17. Davidson, S.J. Emergency unit autotransfusion. *Surgery* 84:703–707, 1978.

18. Mattox, K.L. Comparison of techniques of autotransfusion. *Surgery* 84:700–702, 1978.

19. Noon, G.P. Intraoperative autotransfusion. *Surgery* 84:719–721, 1978.

20. Symbas, P.N. Extraoperative autotransfusion from hemothorax. *Surgery* 84:722–727, 1978.

21. Maughon, J.S. An inquiry into the nature of wounds resulting in killed in action in Vietnam. *Milit Med.* 135:8–13, 1970.

22. *Emergency War Surgery.* U.S. Armed Forces Issue of NATO Handbook. Prepared for use by the Medical Services of NATO Nations. Washington, D.C.: U.S. Government Printing Office, 1958, p. 18.

23. Yates, J.L. Wounds of the chest. Edited by Weld. In *Surgery* Vol. XI, Chap. 14, Medical Department of the U.S. Army in the World War. Washington, D.C.: U.S. Government Printing Office, 1927.

24. Fischer, R.P., Geiger, J.P., and Guernsey, J.M. Pulmonary resections for severe pulmonary contusions secondary to high velocity missile wounds. J Trauma. 14:293–302, 1974.

25. Harvey, E.N., McMillan, J.H., Butler, E.G. et al. Mechanisms of wounding. Edited by J.B. Coates. *Wound Ballistics.* Medical Department of the U.S. Army. Washington, D.C.: U.S. Government Printing Office, 1962, p. 143.

26. DeMuth, W.E. High velocity bullet wounds of the thorax. *Am J Surg.* 115:616–625, 1968.

27. Arom, K.V., Grover, F.L., Richardson, J.D. et al. Posttraumatic empyema. *Ann Thorac Surg.* 23:254–258, 1977.

28. Urschel, H.C., and Razzuk, M.A. Management of acute traumatic injuries of tracheobronchial tree. *Surg Gynecol Obstet.* 136:113–117, 1973.

29. Hodes, P.J., Johnson, J., and Atkins, J.P. Traumatic bronchial rupture with occlusion. *Am J Roentgenol.* 60:448–459, 1948.

30. Holinger, P.H., Zoss, A.R., and Johnston, K.C. Rupture of bronchus due to external chest trauma: report of three cases with recovery. *Laryngoscope* 58:817–833, 1948.

31. Webb, W.R., and Burford, T.H. Studies of the re-expanded lung after prolonged atelectasis. *Arch Surg.* 66:801–809, 1953.

32. Ecker, R.R., Libertini, R.V., Rea, W.J. et al. Injuries of the trachea and bronchi. *Ann Thorac Surg.* 11:289–298, 1971.

33. Grover, F.L., Richardson, J.D., Fewel, J.G. et al. Prophylactic antibiotics in the treatment of penetrating chest wounds: a prospective double-blind study. *J Thorac Cardiovasc Surg.* 74:528–536, 1977.

34. Virgilio, R.W. Intrathoracic wounds in battle casualties. *Surg Gynecol Obstet.* 130:609–615, 1970.

35. Bryant, L.R. Discussion of "Prophylactic antibiotics in the treatment of penetrating chest wounds: A prospective double-blind study." *J Thorac Cardiovasc Surg.* 74:535–536, 1977.

36. *Surgery in World War II.* Vol. I: *Thoracic Surgery.* Washington, D.C.: Office of the Surgeon General, Department of the Army, 1963.

37. Trinkle, J.K., Toon, R.S., Franz, J.L. et al. Affairs of the wounded heart: penetrating cardiac wounds. *J Trauma.* 19:467–472, 1979.

38. Breaux, E.P., Dupont, J.B., Albert, H.M. et al. Cardiac tamponade following penetrating mediastinal injuries: improved survival with early pericardiocentesis. *J Trauma.* 19:461–472, 1979.

39. Evans, J., Gray, L.A., Rayner, A. et al. Principles for the management of penetrating cardiac wounds. *Ann Surg.* 189:777–784, 1979.

40. Sugg, W.L., Rea, W.J., Ecker, R.R. et al. Penetrating wounds of the heart: An analysis of 459 cases. *J Thorac Cardiovasc Surg.* 56:531–543, 1968.

41. Von Berg, V.J., Moggi, L., Jacobson, L.F. et al. Ten years' experience with penetrating injuries of the heart. *J Trauma.* 1:186–194, 1961.

42. Metcalfe, J., Woodbury, J.W., Richards, V. et al. Studies in experimental pericardial tamponade: effects on intravascular pressures and cardiac output. *Circulation* 5:518–523, 1952.

43. Wilson, R.F., and Bassett, J.S. Penetrating wounds of the pericardium and its contents. *JAMA.* 195:513–518, 1966.

44. Yao, S.T., Vanecko, R.M., Printen, K. et al. Penetrating wounds of the heart: a review of 80 cases. *Ann Surg.* 168:67–78, 1968.

45. Lyons, C., and Perkins, R. Cardiac stab wounds. *Am Surg.* 23:507–519, 1957.

46. Larrey, D.J. Clinique chirurgicale, exercée particulièrement dans les camps et les hôpitaux militaires, depuis 1792 jusqu'en 1836. *Paris, Gabon,* 1829–36.

47. Kuno, Y. The mechanical effect of fluid in the pericardium on the function of the heart. *J Physiol.* 51:221–234, 1917.

48. Blalock, A., and Ravitch, M.M. A consideration of the nonoperative treatment of cardiac tamponade resulting from wounds of the heart. *Surgery* 14:157–162, 1943.

49. Elkin, D.C., and Campbell, R.E. Cardiac tamponade: treatment by aspiration. *Ann Surg.* 133:623–630, 1951.

50. Beall, A.C., Diethrich, E.B., Crawford H.W., et al. Surgical management of penetrating cardiac injuries. *Am J Surg.* 112:686–692, 1966.

51. Naclerio, E.A. Penetrating wounds of the heart: experience with 249 patients. *Dis Chest.* 46:1–22, 1964.

52. Maynard, A.L., Cordice, J.W.V., and Naclerio, E.A. Penetrating wounds of the heart: a report of 81 cases. *Surg Gynecol Obstet.* 94:605–618, 1952.

53. Cosman, B., Byerly, W.G., and Wichern, W.A. Penetrating wound of the heart with delayed recurrent hemothorax: case report. *Ann Surg.* 147:87–92, 1958.

54. Mason, L.B., Warshauer, S.E., and Williams, R.W. Stab wound of the heart with delayed hemopericardium. *J Thorac Surg.* 29:524–527, 1955.

55. Pomerantz, M., and Hutchison, D. Traumatic wounds of the heart. *J Trauma.* 9:135–139, 1969.

56. Yao, S.T., Carey, J.S., Shoemaker, W.C. et al. Hemodynamics and therapy of acute hemopericardium from stab wounds of the heart. *J Trauma.* 7:783–792, 1967.

118

57. Sherman, M.M., Saini, V.K., Yarnoz, M.D. et al. Management of penetrating heart wounds. *Am J Surg.* 135:553–558, 1978.

58. Baker, C.C., Thomas, A.N., and Trunkey, D.D. The role of emergency room thoracotomy in trauma. *J Trauma.* (In press). Presented at the 39th Annual Meeting of the American Association for the Surgery of Trauma. Chicago, September 13–15, 1979.

59. Rushforth, N.B., Ford, A.B., Hirsch, C.S. et al. Violent death in a metropolitan county: changing patterns in homicide, 1958–74. *N Engl J Med.* 297:531–538, 1977.

60. Laws, H.L., and Waldschmidt, M.L. Injuries of the diaphragm. *J Trauma.* (In press). Presented at the 39th Annual Meeting of the American Association for the Surgery of Trauma. Chicago, September 13–15, 1979.

7 The Abdomen

In the general treatment of penetrating wounds of the abdomen by gunshot, the surgeon can do little more than to soothe and relieve the patient by the administration of opiates and to treat symptoms of inflammation when they arise on the same principle as in all other cases.*

Gunshot wounds of the abdomen are considerably less lethal than those of the head or thorax. This was very evident in data from the Korean and Vietnam Wars in which fatalities from abdominal wounds were only one-fourth as frequent as those from wounds of the head or thorax.[1,2] The higher fatality rate in head wounds compared to abdominal wounds derives in part from the loss of regulation of respiration and circulation consequent to direct injury to the brain stem, or indirect injury to the brain stem due to displacement or herniation of the brain. The greater lethality of thoracic wounds compared to that of abdominal wounds, depends on at least three pathophysiologic

---

*Longmore, T. *Gunshot Wounds.* Philadelphia: J.B. Lippincott Co., 1863.

phenomena: (1) rapidly fatal hemorrhage from the heart or failure of the heart as a pump; (2) given the ready compressibility of the lungs, the more rapid hemorrhage into pleural cavities compared to the abdominal cavity; (3) the possibility of tracheobronchial injury leading to asphyxia through bilateral pneumothorax. Also contributing to these differences in fatality rates is that in the latter, skeletal injury is less likely. Hence, the dissipation of kinetic energy of the missile and the chances of creating secondary missiles will be substantially less. Although the opportunity for contamination is greater in abdominal wounds, antibiotics and modern surgical debridement and exteriorization of bowel now reduce the fatality rate from abdominal wounds far below the hopeless situation of a century ago.

DIAGNOSIS

Of immediate and major concern, after establishing the track of the bullet and evaluating the stability of the circulatory, respiratory, and nervous systems, is whether the peritoneum has been penetrated and whether the peritoneal cavity should be explored.

Although some disagree, we believe all gunshot wounds of the abdomen should undergo surgical exploration of the peritoneal cavity. The reported experience with gunshot wounds of the abdomen is that more than two-thirds of such patients have intraabdominal injury requiring surgical repair. For example, of 362 patients with gunshot wounds of the abdomen admitted to the Cook County Hospital in Chicago,[3] 70% required surgical repair of intraabdominal structures. Of those patients judged preoperatively to have peritoneal penetration, 98% required surgical repair. Compared to this experience with gunshot wounds, the incidence of such injury from abdominal stab wounds is only 31%, and in those with peritoneal penetration, 80%.[3]

Evidence for peritoneal penetration can be developed from both clinical and laboratory observations. In contrast to the pleural cavity, where the presence of blood does not usually cause pain, blood in the peritoneal cavity elicits a marked chemical peritonitis, abdominal pain, tenderness, and even rebound tenderness. This symptom and these signs may also develop following entry of bile, pancreatic juice, or gastrointestinal contents into the peritoneal cavity. Blood draining from the nasogastric tube or the catheter in the urinary bladder is an obvious indication for abdominal exploration, as is evisceration of abdominal organs. The structure most frequently eviscerating through a relatively small penetrating injury is the omentum (Figures 7-1-7-5). Other evidence for peritoneal penetration is the presence of a metallic foreign body in the abdominal cavity, as indicated by anterior-posterior and lateral radiograms. Other evidence is a hole in the diaphragm observed during thoracotomy. This observation demands exploratory laparotomy. (The reverse is not true. Finding a hole in the diaphragm on exploratory laparotomy is not in itself an indication for thoracotomy; but, this finding does demand immediate tube thoracostomy.)

Peritoneal penetration can, of course, be ascertained surgically. Those who recommend laparotomy only when peritoneal penetration is proved, recommend such exploration of the wound under local anesthesia in the emergency room or under general anesthesia during the management of other injuries. Probing of the wound has been advocated, but is attended with such a high incidence of false-negative results as to contraindicate its use in evaluating the abdominal wound and the indication for laparotomy. The "stabagram" has proven a useful tool. It is based upon demonstrating by a lateral radiogram the appearance of radiopaque contrast material injected through a small catheter placed in the abdominal wound and sutured in place so as to make a watertight seal with the skin. There is a disadvantage in this procedure. Since the contrast material is irritating because of its hyperosmolarity, it will cause localized pain and tenderness and may produce a wound abscess if it remains confined to the somatic structures, as would be the case if there is not a hole in the peritoneum. The material does not irritate the peritoneum, however, because it is absorbed rapidly.

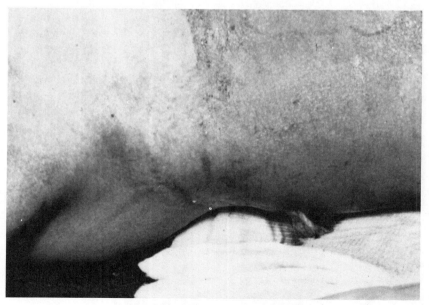

Figure 7-1 A 12-year-old male sustained an AK-47 gunshot wound of the left flank during a firefight. He had a single wound of entrance from which herniated a small piece of omentum. No exit wound was observed.

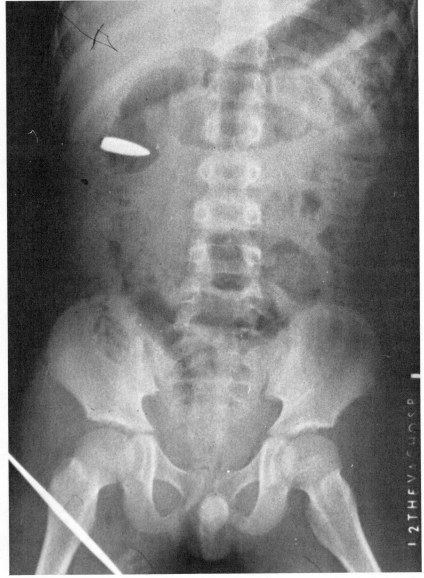

Figure 7-2 An A-P radiogram view of the abdomen reveals a bullet in the region of the right upper quadrant.

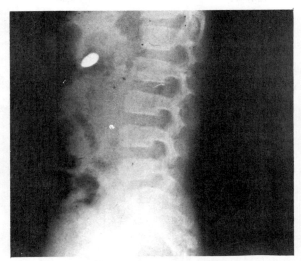

Figure 7-3 A lateral radiogram confirms the probable presence of the round within the abdomen. Thus, two indications for abdominal exploration are present: (1) evisceration, and (2) metallic foreign body within the abdomen.

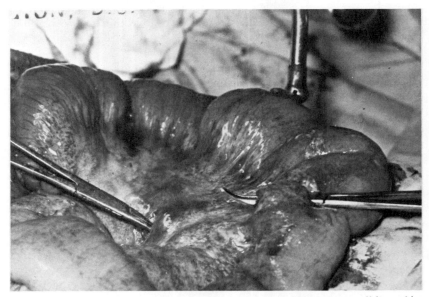

Figure 7-4 Surgical exploration reveals multiple holes in the small bowel as identified by the curved clamp and the suction tip. The round is located within the small bowel mesentery and is identified by the needle holder. Small-bowel resection was carried out because of the proximity of multiple holes in the small bowel and because of the location of one wound on the mesenteric border of the bowel, which thus subjected the patient to further threat of ischemic injury because of the proximity of the wound to the blood supply of the bowel wall. An injured transverse colon was also identified.

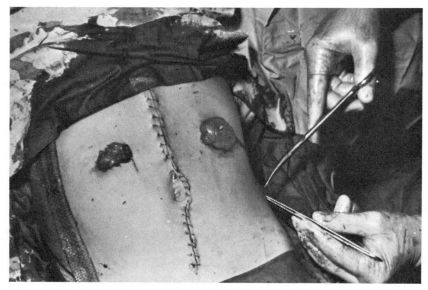

Figure 7-5 The patient's abdomen has been closed; the colon injury was treated with a double-barreled colostomy wth a skin bridge between the (proximal) colostomy and the (distal) mucous fistula. The skin incision could have been left open and undergone delayed primary closure within one week's time. The entrance wound is being debrided.

Radioactive scanning of the liver and spleen may reveal the presence of parenchymal rupture or intracapsular hematoma, particularly in the case of the spleen. Selective arteriography may be useful in demonstrating injury to liver, spleen, or kidney. These methods are not always available in most institutions on a 24-hour basis, and probably at the present time, do not warrant inclusion in the armamentarium of the physician managing a penetrating abdominal injury. Sonography and computerized axial tomography will undoubtedly come into use in the more precise localization of intraabdominal gunshot wounds.

Perhaps the simplest of all diagnostic tests, but the one that is most frequently omitted in the management of a patient with possible penetrating abdominal injury, is the rectal examination. Rarely is the left side of the colon injured without gross blood being identified on digital examination of the rectum. Although proctoscopy probably should be performed whenever blood is found within the rectum following abdominal or perineal trauma, it is rarely informative. In all likelihood all that will be found on proctosigmoidoscopy is more blood and stool. In a gunshot wound including the trunk or thighs, finding blood in the rectum in the face of negative proctosigmoidoscopy and exploratory laparotomy, mandates a diverting sigmoid colostomy.

Peritoneal lavage is an increasingly popular technique for evaluating the acute abdomen. The technique is applicable to wounds of the abdomen and chest.[4,5] The technique has proven highly effective (95% accuracy), showing low incidences of false-positive (3%) and false-negative (2%) results. A contraindication to peritoneal lavage is the presence of an abdominal scar and the likelihood of adhesions, making hollow viscera vulnerable to perforation during paracentesis.

In peritoneal lavage, a small infraumbilical incision is made under local anesthesia. The linea alba is incised, and a 1-cm incision is made in the peritoneum. An ordinary peritoneal dialysis unit and its peritoneal catheter are utilized for the test. The catheter is inserted into the peritoneal cavity, and a liter of isotonic (0.9%) saline, 5% dextrose in water, or preferably Ringer's lactate solution is infused. The fluid is permitted sufficient time to distribute within the peritoneal cavity; changing the patient's position assists in this. Depending upon the patient's condition, the fluid is drained from the peritoneal cavity 5 to 30 minutes later. Normally, approximately 750 ml can be recovered. If the fluid is grossly pink, if ordinary newspaper print cannot be read through a test tube containing the fluid, or if the fluid contains in excess of 50,000 to 100,000 red blood cells per mm^3 of test fluid, the lavage is considered positive. Obviously, if there is gross bleeding from the peritoneal cavity through the incision, then the test is positive, and lavage is not performed. As Lucas[4] has emphasized, the incidence of false-negative lavage is small, but present in all series reported. If suspicion persists regarding intraabdominal injury attending gunshot wounds, a negative lavage should not deter laparotomy.

MANAGEMENT

Once surgery is decided upon, the patient's preoperative preparation should include the availability of whole blood and, depending upon age and general preoperative condition, an assessment of plasma electrolyte and arterial blood gas concentrations. Preoperative antibiotic therapy is probably indicated, but evidence for its value is meager, despite the long-standing debate regarding prophylactic antibiotic therapy in penetrating abdominal trauma. For optimal effectiveness antibiotics probably should be administered during the inital resuscitation period, continued through the operative procedure, and, depending upon the operative findings, continued for 24 hours postoperatively. Systemic venous access in both upper and lower extremities is desirable, particularly if there is question of major injury to veins of the trunk. Most surgeons would agree that the best exposure for management of intraabdominal trauma is a midline incision extending, if necessary, from the xiphoid to the pubis. Experience also teaches that the entire abdomen, as well as the chest and the anterior thighs, should be included in the sterile field so as to permit access to the thorax, or the saphenous vein for autogenous graft.

Once the peritoneal cavity has been entered, it is important to eviscerate promptly the small bowel and tranverse colon so as to assess quickly the contained injury. This improves exposure and enables identification of retroperitoneal hematomata, splenic and hepatic injury, diaphragmatic injury, and other sources of major hemorrhage. For obvious reasons, control of hemorrhage takes precedence over other concerns. As elsewhere in the management of trauma, an orderly assessment of priorities and their appropriate management is imperative if disaster is to be averted or, conversely, success anticipated.

The Spleen

Solitary splenic injuries are rarely a therapeutic dilemma for the surgeon, since they are readily resolved with splenectomy. An orderly, urgent splenectomy requires mobilization of the spleen, which in turn involves sharp dissection of the parietal peritoneal attachments of this organ. These consist of the lienorenal and lienophrenic ligaments. This procedure facilitates mobilization of the spleen into the operative field, so that its pedicle can be serially cross-clamped, divided, and ligated. Medium (2-0) silk is appropriate for this phase of the splenectomy, primarily to avoid suture breakage and escape of important blood vessels from the operative field. Generous use of suture ligation (3-0 silk) is wise if not excessively time-consuming. Dividing the splenic pedicle close to the spleen minimizes possible injury to the tail of the pancreas. Such an injury complicates a significant percentage of emergency splenectomies. Recent information indicates that in children, adolescents, and perhaps even young adults, the spleen is an important organ in terms of minimizing systemic infections which might attend penetrating injuries of the abdominal cavity at the time of the initial assault, or which might occur subsequent to recovery. Because of the growing understanding of the role of the spleen in immunity, splenectomy for control of hemorrhage is being undertaken less cavalierly, especially in younger individuals. However, concern about immunity should not take precedence over hemostasis. Techniques such as suture ligation, Gelfoam, topical thrombogenic agents, etc., have all been utilized successfully in controlling bleeding from minor splenic injuries.

Although every effort should be made to preserve the spleen in the younger age group, it should be recognized that late complications of splenic injury do exist. Pseudocysts may accompany splenic injury, may subsequently enlarge to gigantic proportions, and eventually require surgery.[6] These cysts may undergo relatively rapid growth and present within months after initial injury as a complaint of increasing abdominal girth.[6,7] In addition, delayed rupture of the spleen has been reported as late as five years following the initial injury.[8] Such a delay is a rare pathological event, and it is generally held that 75% of delayed ruptures of the spleen occur within the first two weeks after injury, and 90% within the first four weeks.[9] In fact, delayed rupture of the spleen is often thought to represent delayed recognition of splenic injury.[10] Approximately 75% of patients with a splenic injury complain of pain in the left shoulder (Kehr sign).[8,11] Occasionally shoulder pain is bilateral.[8]

If time permits, celiac angiography is an excellent technique for diagnosing injuries to the spleen, and yields a very low incidence of false-positive or false-negative results.[12] Conversely, splenic scanning, although a more easily accomplished diagnostic procedure than angiography, suffers from the fact that nonspecific defects are diagnosed; that is, other nontraumatic conditions such as splenic cyst may simulate a traumatic injury.[13] The diagnosis of splenic injury is important because its neglect carries a 90% to 95% mortality.[14] Isolated but treated injury to the spleen carries a relatively low mortality rate (1%).[15] Conversely, splenic injury associated with injury to other viscera carries a relatively high mortality rate (in the neighborhood of 18%).[16]

One of the yet unresolved questions with regard to emergency splenectomy for the management of traumatic splenic injury concerns utilization of drains to the splenic bed. Perhaps the most common complication attending emergency splenectomy, regardless of the indication, is left subphrenic abscess. This complication and its prophylactic, as well as therapeutic, management continue to challenge the surgeon. Assuming no obvious source of intraperitoneal contamination, such as injury to hollow viscus, and assuming an emergency splenectomy with adequate hemostasis, theoretically no indication exists for prophylactic drainage of the left subphrenic space. Yet, if there is coexistent injury to the large bowel, small bowel, stomach, or even pancreas, there is a good chance for secondary infection culminating in a subphrenic abscess following emergency splenectomy. The best approach to this potential threat is prophylactic drainage, but the duration of the drainage is debatable. Should the drains be of relatively brief (48 to 72 hours) duration, which would minimize the subphrenic accumulation of those fluids potentiating a subphrenic abscess? Should the drains be left for a longer time (seven to ten days) to drain therapeutically an anticipated subphrenic abscess? We personally favor the latter course of surgical management, which realistically anticipates the abscess as though it were imminent. Sump-tube drainage is appropriate under these circumstances, but the sump tube is literally a "two-edged sword"; if left in place for more than 72 hours, there exists the risk of perforation of hollow viscus because of the relatively rigid nature of even the softest of sump tubes. Two large Penrose drains, passed through a stab wound that admits two fingers, probably best adequately drain the left subphrenic space. Preferably, the drains exit through a posterolateral stab wound, optimizing dependency. This stab wound can be easily made with a scalpel blade from inside the peritoneal cavity and passed exteriorly. The scalpel blade is then met externally with a Kelly clamp, reintroduced, and replaced with Penrose drains that are then brought from inside the peritoneal cavity externally. This procedure is consistent with the suggested practice of externalizing drains from inside the peritoneal cavity to minimize the risk of contamination from the skin.

The Liver

The management of penetrating hepatic injuries does not differ significantly from the management of blunt trauma to the liver. Three alternatives are available for surgical attempts at hemostasis: (1) drainage, (2) suture ligation, and (3) partial resection. Whereas relatively minor injuries to the spleen are usually treated by splenectomy, relatively minor injuries to the liver can be tolerated if drainage is appropriately exteriorized. Thus, minimal amounts of bleeding from a relatively small hepatic laceration can be managed without suture ligation or resection, if the area is appropriately drained so that the intraperitoneal accumulation of blood and bile can be appropriately externalized. Stellate lacerations of the liver, whether due to blunt trauma or to through-and-through gunshot wounds, require more extensive surgical maneuvers. One of these is the Pringle maneuver.[17,18] This consists of encircling the portal triad (proper hepatic artery, portal vein, and common bile duct) with either a Penrose drain or a noncrushing (vascular) clamp, resulting in cessation of blood flow to the liver.[18,19] The only source of bleeding from the injured liver is thus limited to the hepatic venous side of the hepatic circulation. If the surgeon is standing on the left side of the patient's body, this maneuver is executed by inserting the left index finger into the foramen of Winslow and approximating thumb and index finger through the lesser omentum, thus encircling the portal triad and guiding the application of a clamp or tourniquet to these structures. This maneuver probably will cause a dramatic diminution in bleeding from the injured liver. This occlusion can be safely maintained without hepatic damage for ten to 15 minutes under normothermic conditions and even longer if the patient is hypothermic.[18,20,21] Often, this procedure will enable the surgeon to mobilize more adequately his reserves in terms of whole blood replacement, operating team, surgical exposure, etc.

If the injury to the liver is confined to the left lobe, a left hepatic lobectomy is easily accomplished. Conversely, a right hepatic lobectomy usually requires thoracoabdominal exposure of the right lobe and its venous drainage. Traditionally, a right thoracotomy has accompanied the midline abdominal incision, but some have advocated a median sternotomy to give equally adequate, and perhaps more advantageous, exposure.* Right hepatic lobectomy is a relatively formidable procedure which carries a mortality in excess of 50%.[19] With division of the right hemidiaphragm, the critical structures can be identified; these include the hepatic veins and vena cava. An anatomic resection of the right lobe of the liver involves dissection just lateral to, but may include, the gallbladder.[18] The finger fracture technique of Lin is probably the most expeditious technique of hepatic resection; however, alternative techniques such as use of the Doty clamp have been successfully employed. The use of prophylactic, common bile-duct drainage has been largely abandoned, despite the fact that many have championed its use in the past. At the present time, it is considered inappropriate to attempt cannulation of a healthy, common bile duct of normal diameter.

In a series of 546 cases of hepatic injury in civil life the vast majority (85%) of which were due to penetrating injuries, of which gunshot wounds constituted two-thirds of the injuries, there was only a 5% mortality if the liver was the only organ injured.[19] When hepatic injury was accompanied by injury to other organs, the mortality rate doubled (10%).

Overall mortality for stab wounds was negligible (0.6%), and interestingly, patients sustaining gunshot wounds incurred less than half the mortality (12%) than those whose injury was caused by blunt trauma (28%). When the penetrating wound was secondary to high-velocity wounds including shotgun blasts at close range, the hepatic injury simulated that secondary to blunt trauma, thus putting these two categories of wounds (gunshot wounds and blunt trauma) into the same category with regard to diagnosis, treatment, and prognosis. Whether the injury is due to blunt trauma or to high-velocity missile injury, the mortality will be high and will approach two-thirds if hepatectomy is required.[20,21]

Abdominal tenderness is the most common presenting complaint in liver injury and appears in 70% of patients.[19] Most patients with liver injury (70%) have more than one organ involved in the injury, the diaphragm, stomach, and colon being the other organs most frequently injured.[19] One or the other of these three organs is injured in approximately 20% of cases of hepatic injury. The kidney, spleen, pancreas, and small bowel are the next most commonly injured organs, one or the other damaged in 10% of patients with hepatic injury.[19] The overall

---

*G. Tom Shires, personal communication, 1978.

mortality rate for hepatic lobectomy is over 50%.[19-21] In the series of hepatic injuries referred to above,[19,21] the mortality from stab wounds was 0.6%; that from gunshot wounds, 12%, and from blunt trauma, 25%. When the firearm was a shotgun, mortality was more than twice as high as with other types of guns. Nearly all of the patients were managed by compression suture, drainage, and debridement,[19] with a low mortality (7.6%) resulting. The remaining 6% of the cases required formal hepatic lobectomy, with a resultant mortality of 52%.

Although the small bowel is most commonly injured when the source of trauma is penetrating injury,[22] and the spleen is the organ most frequently injured when the trauma is blunt,[23] when blunt and penetrating abdominal trauma are combined, the organ most commonly involved is the liver.[19] The major cause of death in hepatic trauma is hemorrhage. In another large series of hepatic injuries,[24] only 11% required a major procedure for control of hemorrhage. Hepatic lobectomy, with mortality in excess of 50%, obviously carries an ominous prognosis.[20,21,25,26]

Hepatic arterial ligation has been advocated for the control of massive hepatic injury and has been successful in some hands.[18] In an adolescent the proper hepatic artery has been ligated successfuly in the management of bilobar hepatic trauma and with minimal and transient hepatic dysfunction.[27] Others have been less successful with the use of this procedure in the management of hepatic trauma,[24] and this result has led some[19] to advocate hepatic arterial ligation only when alternative techniques have failed to control hemorrhage or have been impracticable.

One of the most difficult forms of hepatic injury with which to deal is that related to injuries involving the hepatic vein and retrohepatic vena cava. These injuries are evidenced by continued venous bleeding from the liver, despite occlusion of the portal triad. Vascular isolation of the liver, as described by Schrock in 1968,[28] involves shunting of blood from the infrahepatic inferior vena cava to the right atrium and can be accomplished with readily available materials such as a chest tube or Foley catheter. A relatively simple technique involves insertion of a large-bore chest tube through a pursestring suture around a right atriotomy. The chest tube is fenestrated at its atrial level before insertion and clamped at its cardiac external level. An occlusive ligature is tied around the suprarenal inferior vena cava containing the other end of the chest tube. This allows inferior vena caval blood to return to the heart through the chest tube, bypassing the hepatic venous injury. The inferior vena cava is also ligated about the chest tube above the diaphragm to isolate the vena cava in the region of the hepatic venous injury.

High-velocity gunshot wounds, which include shotgun injuries sustained at close range, produce extensive damage to the liver and simulate the bursting stellate laceration of the liver characteristic of blunt abdominal trauma.[29] Development of hemobilia[30] following repair of liver injury suggests that the initial operative procedure was inadequate and that the patient will require additional surgery and debridement of the damaged liver.[29]

The Gallbladder

Injury to the gallbladder is probably best managed with cholecystectomy, since attempts at suture repair of injuries to this structure are considered to result in probable nidi for gallstone formation. Injury to the common bile duct is best treated with primary repair utilizing fine, absorbable suture material (although this too is controversial) over a T-tube for decompression.

The Portal Venous System

Injury to the portal venous system (portal vein, superior mesenteric vein, splenic vein, and inferior mesenteric vein) carries a mortality of 33%. A typical case requires about 12 units of blood[31] (Figures 7-6–7-10).

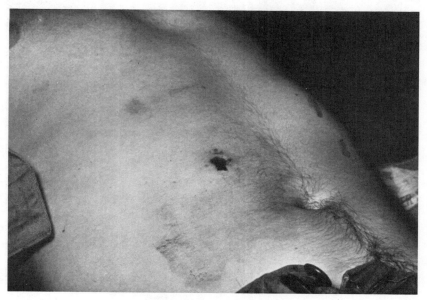

Figure 7-6 A 19-year-old soldier sustained a fragment wound of the abdomen from a hand grenade. He had a single entrance wound within the right upper abdominal quadrant. There was tenderness and rebound tenderness on abdominal examination.

132

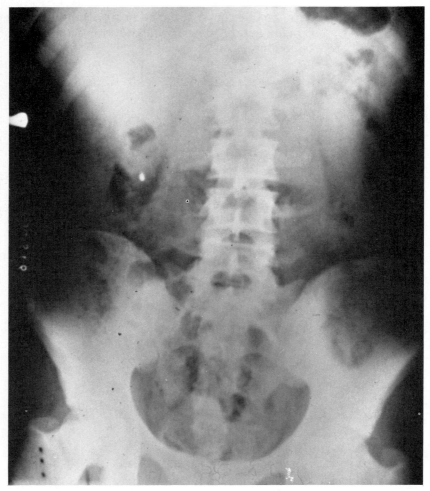

Figure 7-7 Abdominal radiogram (A-P view) reveals a metallic foreign body in the right side of the abdomen.

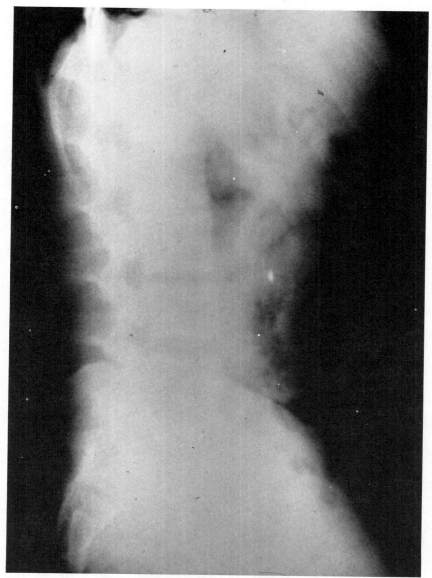

Figure 7-8 Lateral radiogram of the abdomen confirms the probable presence of the fragment within the abdomen. Thus, there are two indications for abdominal exploration: (1) positive physical findings on abdominal exam, and (2) presence of a metallic foreign body within the abdomen.

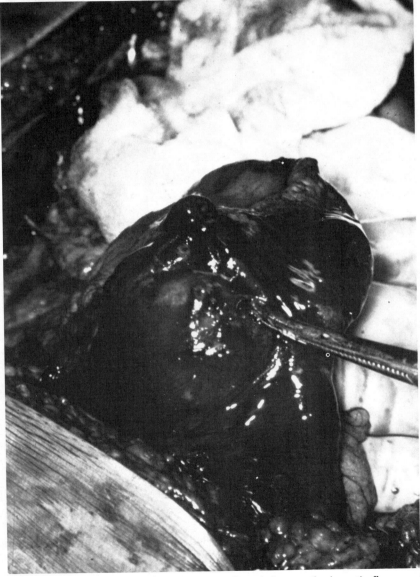

Figure 7-9 Abdominal exploration reveals an injury to the hepatic flexure of the colon (identified by the curved clamp).

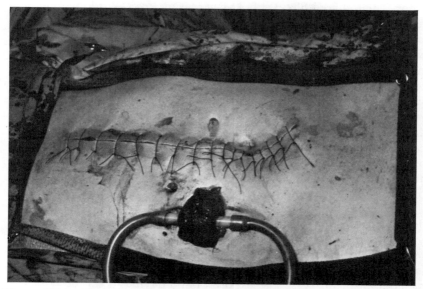

Figure 7-10 The injured colon was exteriorized as a colostomy; the entrance wound was debrided. The abdominal incision could have been left open to await delayed primary closure if necessitated by significant fecal contamination observed at surgery.

The Stomach

Penetrating injuries of the stomach are readily managed with suture ligation to accomplish hemostasis related to bleeding from the gastric mucosa, followed by serosal repair utilizing interrupted, fine, nonabsorbable sutures. Silk (3-0) is entirely appropriate for this maneuver. The surgeon should "take down" the greater curvature of the stomach in order to examine adequately its posterior surface for injury. This maneuver also enables direct examination of the pancreas.

Clear nasogastric tube drainage is not inconsistent with through-and-through penetration of the stomach from a gunshot wound. Partial or even total gastrectomy is an appropriate method of managing extensive injury to the stomach. Gastrostomy for decompression is not contraindicated in the management of penetrating injuries of the stomach, but does jeopardize any suture line in the surgical repair of such injuries. Usually, nasogastric tube decompression of·the stomach is sufficient.

The Pancreas and Duodenum

The intimate anatomic relations between the duodenum and pancreas frequently result in a gunshot wound of one organ involving the other. Their shared blood supply is a reason why debridement and/or resection of one may require resection of the other, even though the latter is intact.[32] The potential difficulty of management is evident when one considers that surgical repair may even require radical pancreaticoduodenectomy (the Whipple procedure). Mortality with this procedure, as an elective operation, approaches 20% and probably is substantially higher when it is performed on an emergency basis and when the caliber of the common bile duct is normal. Adding to the danger of such a gunshot wound is the proximity of the aorta and vena cava, and the fact that the morbidity and the incidence of late complications of surgery in this region are high. Thus, upon opening the abdomen the trauma surgeon views with dismay an injury to the pancreas or duodenum.

An injury limited to the tail of the pancreas is readily managed by debridement and/or partial resection and drainage. Because of the proximity of the tail of the pancreas to the spleen, injury to the latter, or its pedicle, may require splenectomy. The pancreatic duct should be identified and ligated to reduce the chance of pancreatic fistula, pseudocyst or abscess. The exposed parenchyma of the body of the pancreas should be closed with mattress sutures. Whether these sutures should be absorbable or not is moot.

In American civil life today, the most common traumatic injury to the duodenum is a penetrating injury, and that is most commonly a gunshot wound.[32] Because of the proximity of the duodenum to the aorta and vena cava, many victims of gunshot wounds of the duodenum die before reaching the hospital. Among patients with duodenal wounds who come to surgery, injury to the vena cava is the most commonly associated lesion. The other organs most frequently injured in association with a wound of the duodenum are the colon, liver, stomach, and as mentioned above, the pancreas.[32] The second portion of the duodenum is the most commonly injured part.[33]

In contrast to wounds involving the urinary tract and other parts of the gastrointestinal tract, other than the apparent path of the projectile, there is little preoperative evidence obtainable to define injury to the duodenum. Such injuries are usually only ascertained by laparotomy. In a few patients, radiogram of the abdomen may reveal obliteration of the right psoas shadow, scoliosis (concavity to the right), or gas under the diaphragm. Leakage of water-soluble radiopaque contrast material introduced through a nasogastric tube, can confirm the diagnosis. Regardless of the radiographic findings, laparotomy is necessary. If the perforation of the duodenum is small and less than six hours old, it should be closed primarily. Transverse closure is preferred, since longitudinal closure is more likely to compromise the lumen. Proximal drainage via the nasogastric tube may be insufficient. For this reason, some[32] recommend supplementing primary closure with proximal drainage by a duodenostomy, or gastrostomy. After six hours, tube drainage through the defect ("controlled duodenostomy") and, depending upon the relative size of the defect, closure of the bowel around the tube are recommended.[32] Complications of primary closure include duodenal or pancreatic fistulae and abdominal sepsis.[33,34,35]

When the injury to the duodenum is more extensive than a simple perforation, diverticulization[36] involving, of course, transection of the pylorus and gastrojejunostomy,[32] may be required. If the injury is extensive and localized to the third or fourth parts of the duodenum, resection and end-to-end anastomosis may be possible. This is not an option in more proximal duodenal injuries because of the presence of the common bile duct and the duodenal blood supply shared with the head of the pancreas.[32] To diminish gastric secretion and its deleterious effect on the suture line, pyloroplasty and vagotomy at the time of duodenal closure, have been advocated.[33] The "three tube" approach, i.e., afferent jejunostomy for decompression, efferent jejunostomy for feeding, and gastrostomy for decompression proximal to the duodenal repair,[32,33] has also been recommended as minimizing the development of a duodenal fistula or marginal ulcer complicating a gastrojejunostomy. In an extensive, ragged, or old duodenal injury, the serosal or omental patch technique can be applied.[32,33] In even more extensive duodenal wounds, especially those involving the second part, formal pancreaticoduodenectomy may be required.[32]

Appropriate application of primary closure of a duodenal gunshot wound can be expected to lead to recovery in approximately 85% of cases. When there is associated pancreatic injury, mortality doubles.[32,37-40] When closure is delayed beyond 24 hours, duodenal fistula is a much more frequent complication, and mortality quadruples.[41]

The Small Intestine

In gunshot wounds of the abdomen, injury to the jejunum, ileum, and their mesenteries is more frequent than injury to any other intra-abdominal organ. The diagnosis is rarely established preoperatively and even if made, would not alter the surgical approach, but would strengthen the indication for preoperative antibiotic therapy. Radiographic evidence of gas under the diaphragm may be present, but of course may be from other parts of the gastrointestinal tract. At laparotomy, the jejunum and ileum should be eviscerated and carefully inspected from ligament of Treitz to cecum, and any injury marked with a fine black silk suture. The "rule of two"[42] is that an odd number of perforations demands careful search for an additional hole before labeling the odd one a tangential wound.

Injuries to the small intestine are relatively easy to correct surgically. If the defect to the small bowel is on the antemesenteric border, and isolated as well as relatively small, it can be closed with inverting nonabsorbable suture material which approximates serosa. Where segments of bowel are involved with multiple gunshot wounds, resection and end-to-end anastomosis are appropriate. The primary consideration is luminal competency, and this should not be challenged by the nature of the repair. In other words, if luminal competency is compromised as a result of suture plication of an injury to the small bowel, resection is a more acceptable alternative. If the injury to the small bowel is along the mesenteric border (see Figure 7-4), resection should be strongly considered, since primary repair on this border of the small bowel may compromise the vascular integrity of the viscus.

Whenever a penetrating injury to the small bowel is encountered, a careful search should be carried out for possible additional entrance or exit wounds. For obvious reasons, to leave one defect unrepaired, while at the same time repairing numerous others is to condemn the patient to the threat of postoperative peritonitis. When one approaches the distal part of the ileum, stronger consideration should be given to primary repair as opposed to resection, in consideration of the specific function of the distal ileum in bile salt and vitamin B_{12} absorption. Defects in the small bowel do not need to be treated with prophylactic drainage, although this is a somewhat controversial issue. Local application of antibiotics, or antibiotic solutions, as well as irrigation of the peritoneal cavity, are always considerations when there is contamination from penetrating injuries of the small bowel. Our opinion is that neither of these maneuvers will minimize the incidence of postoperative complications.

An exception to the above recommendations is in the case of a shotgun (as distinguished from gunshot) wound in which peritoneal penetration is evident radiographically. If the shot (i.e., pellets) is fine (e.g., No. 9), the number of perforations may be very numerous and very small. The chance of spontaneous closure of such small perforations, as in the case of a needle perforation, justifies the withholding of surgery.

The Colon

Second only to the small intestine, the colon is the most commonly injured intraabdominal viscus following penetrating trauma to the peritoneal cavity. Injuries to additional structures are common, and thus considerations for other than just the injury to the large intestine will influence its management.

The diagnosis is usually not established prior to surgery; however, certain observations should suggest the probability of colonic injury. Blood on the examining finger following rectal examination is diagnostic and, in fact, alone and despite any other positive finding either prior to or at surgery, is an indication for diverting sigmoid colostomy, since rectal injury is implied. An A-P radiogram of the abdomen in the upright position may reveal gas under the diaphragm, but this finding is not specific other than to suggest injury to hollow viscus. Precisely for this reason, however, the radiogram should be obtained prior to peritoneal lavage, since the latter procedure itself may introduce air into the peritoneal cavity. Proctosigmoidoscopy is indicated if digital examination of the rectum reveals blood; however, it must be mentioned that proctosigmoidoscopy is relatively uncommonly contributory to either diagnosis or therapy, since the rectum is obviously unprepared for the procedure. Usually all the examiner observes is more blood and stool; rarely is the specific injury identified. For the same reason, colonoscopy is not likely to prove helpful, and because of the risk of additional injury to the large intestine, is contraindicated in the preoperative evaluation of penetrating abdominal injuries. Barium enema is contraindicated because of the probability of intraperitoneal leak, and the fact that most injuries to the colon (Figures 7-6–7-10), as compared to those of the rectum (Figures 7-11-7-16), are readily apparent at laparotomy.

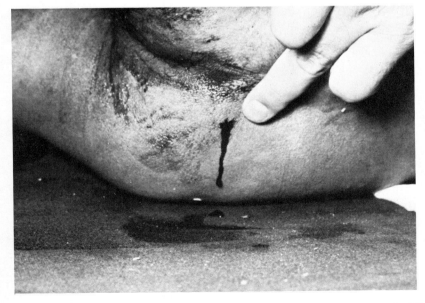

Figure 7-11 A 31-year-old soldier sustained an M-16 gunshot wound of the right buttock from a distance of 150 m. The wound of entrance is identified.

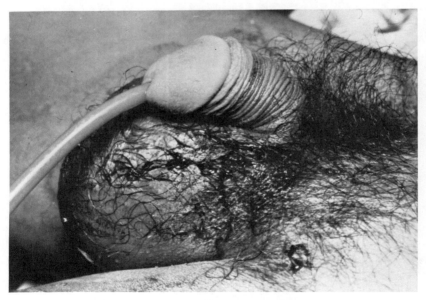

Figure 7-12 A single exit wound is located in the left inguinal region.

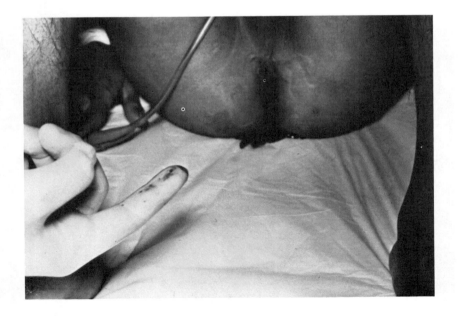

Figure 7-13   Digital examination of the rectum is positive for occult blood.

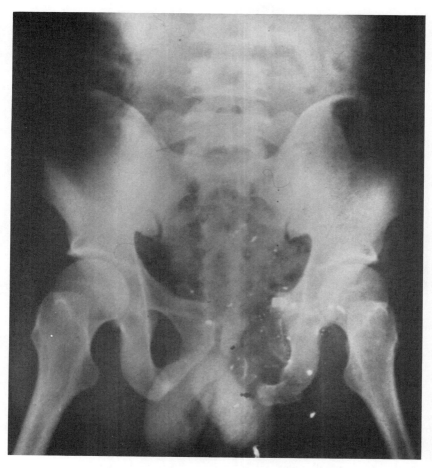

Figure 7-14   Radiographic view (A-P) of the pelvis reveals multiple small metallic foreign bodies and destruction of the superior and inferior pubic rami.

144

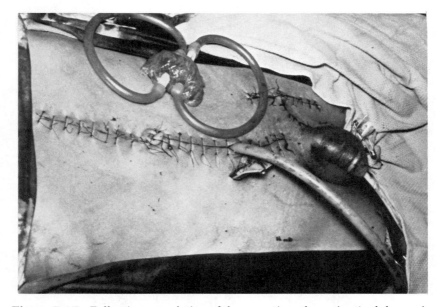

Figure 7-15 Following completion of the operation, the patient's abdomen is viewed to show a sigmoid colostomy indicated by blood on the examining finger during digital examination of the rectum and despite negative proctosigmoidoscopy, abdominal, and pelvic explorations. The left common femoral artery and vein were explored because of their proximity to the exit wound. These vessels were not injured. A cystostomy tube is in place. A Penrose drain is in the prevesical space. A Foley catheter is placed in the bladder transurethrally.

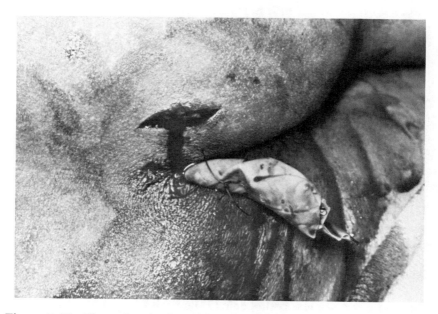

Figure 7-16 The patient is viewed from the position of the entrance wound and lying on his left side. Coccygectomy has been performed, and drains placed in the pelvis at the time of abdominal and pelvic exploration exteriorized. These are prophylactic in nature and aimed at a potential pelvic abscess associated with a presumed rectal injury. The entrance wound has been debrided.

There is as yet no compelling evidence for the value of antibiotics prophylactically in the management of penetrating wounds of the abdomen.[43] Empirical use of these agents has gained wide acceptance. In principle, their value is likely to be greater in injuries of the colon. For this reason, we believe preoperative recognition (blood on rectal examination) of injury indicates immediate antibiotic therapy. Intravenous cephalosporins at a rate of 1 gm every four hours is our current recommendation. Although laparotomy is mandatory in suspected gunshot wounds of the large intestine, subsequent surgical management is controversial. Despite many innovative techniques derived from recent civil and military experience, morbidity and mortality remain high.

A range of surgical procedures is available to the trauma surgeon in operative management of gunshot wounds of the colon and rectum. The number of alternatives attests to the fact that no single procedure has been continually successful. Each has its advantages and disadvantages. Resection and exteriorization with a double-barreled colostomy including a skin bridge between the proximal bowel (colostomy) and the distal bowel (mucous fistula) is the safest initial management of any penetrating injury to the colon. As the Vietnam War proceeded, this procedure became the ultimate choice, reflecting unsatisfactory results with the so-called lesser procedures, including primary repair of right colon wounds. Failure of the latter became generally apparent by 1970, after which double-barreled colostomy became virtually mandated. The reason for rejection of primary repair was the observation that intraabdominal, and usually pelvic, abscess occurred relatively frequently following primary repair of even right colon injuries. The inadequacy of primary colon repair had not been apparent earlier to operating teams in Vietnam because of the policy of early postoperative air evacuation "out of country" had precluded follow-up by operating surgeons.

One must recall that parasympathetic innervation of the ascending and transverse parts of the colon, as well as more proximal parts of the alimentary tract, is vagal, while parasympathetic innervation of the descending and sigmoid colon and rectum is through sacral segments two through four. Several anatomic, physiologic, and microbiologic characteristics correspond to this neural subdivision. The right colon is of relatively large caliber when compared to the colon distal to the splenic flexure. The stool content of the right colon is relatively liquid when compared to that on the left side. The bacterial flora inhabiting the right colon are less pathogenic to the peritoneal cavity than those on the left. The "right colon" (cecum, ascending colon, and transverse colon) has thus been viewed as similar to small bowel in that penetrating injuries to either can be treated in identical fashion under most circumstances. Thus, simple closure or resection and primary anastomosis are procedures which find application to wounds of these parts of the large intestine. Although it ultimately became the policy in Vietnam to treat all wounds of the large intestine by exteriorization, it would seem that under optimal conditions in civilian life some wounds of the right colon can be treated by resection and primary anastomosis, or by simple closure.

Alternative procedures to double-barreled colostomy include primary closure, primary closure and exteriorization, and conversion of the wounded colon to a colostomy. A fourth is the Hartmann procedure, or distal closure and proximal colostomy. The latter is particularly applicable to injuries to the distal left colon and proximal rectum. The basis for selection of the surgical procedure will be viewed in the following historic perspective.

The mortality from colon wounds during World War I was high (60%)[44] and reflected in part the policy of primary closure of the wounds. In World War II, when proximal diverting colostomy or exteriorization, as advocated by Mason,[45] came into use mortality fell to 31%.[46] The Korean War saw a further reduction to 15%,[44] where it remained during the Vietnam War. The recent civilian mortality ranges from 7% to 15%.[43,47-49] Since 75% to 80% of patients with wounds involving the colon have associated injuries to other organs,[47,48] further reduction in the mortality from such wounds can be expected to depend more upon advances in the management of these associated wounds than upon advances in the management of wounds of the colon itself.

The debate between those who favor primary closure of colon injuries and those who advocate exclusion of the injured segment from the fecal stream continues. Some advise primary repair in the case of injury to the right colon[48,50] and diversion for injuries to the left colon.[49] Opponents of this so-called "anatomic approach" to colonic injuries argue that the complication rate associated with repair of injuries to the right colon far exceeds that associated with repair of injuries to the left colon.[43,48,51,52] (It should be recognized that this rate is influenced by the more liberal use of primary closure of right colonic versus left colonic injuries.) We believe the argument depends upon the nature of the wounding agent. Gunshot wounds to the colon carry a higher risk than stab wounds; blunt trauma to the colon is even more threatening.[42,43,50] It also depends upon the interval between wounding and surgery,[42,50] the degree of peritoneal contamination, the quality and quantity of colonic contents, and the extent of associated injuries.

An innovative variation on exteriorization of the colonic injury is primary closure and return of the injured segment (interiorization) six to ten days later, provided the suture line is intact. Although this technique was described during World War II,[45] it has gained little popularity until relatively recently[48] because most surgeons are fearful of poor healing of suture lines in intestine exposed to the air.[53] Experimental evidence[54] suggests that this concern is unjustified. Careful attention to the exposed suture line with constant application of isotonically moist dressings is essential to maintain integrity of the suture line. Another innovation is described by Kirkpatrick[53] consisting of a fascial bridge instead of the usual glass or polyethylene rod. The latter has been traditionally used to prevent the exteriorized segment from falling back into the peritoneal cavity. The fascial bridge is thought to prevent obstruction of the large bowel, which occasionally attends use of the rod, particularly when the exteriorized segment is under tension.

Sigmoid resection and primary anastomosis for gunshot injuries is associated with a high failure. Cecostomy is associated with prolonged delay in spontaneous closure.

Injuries to the rectum mandate proximal diverting colostomy. There is little disagreement on this point. In the past transverse colostomy was often used to divert the fecal stream under such circumstances. It is now generally appreciated that sigmoid colostomy[42] is a more appropriate procedure,[43] since it is as easily accomplished and is closer to the injured segment. We and others[43] believe that the distal colon and rectum should be flushed free of contained stool from "above and below" at the time of surgery. Either a loop-type sigmoid colostomy, or a double-barreled colostomy, or an end colostomy with distal closure (Hartmann procedure), is acceptable.

Colorectal gunshot wounds should be treated with extraperitoneal dissection to the coccyx at the time of laparotomy for the placement of Penrose drains deep in the pelvis prior to pelvic peritoneal and abdominal closure. Following abdominal closure, the patient is turned and coccygectomy performed. The latter procedure enables the surgeon to dissect proximally for a short distance in order to recover the drains for exteriorization. This prophylactic measure provides potential drainage of a possible pelvic abscess. This is a threat whenever the left colon is injured. Since the sacrococcygeal region will probably be the most dependent during the first ten postoperative days it seems reasonable to anticipate further that pus accumulated from intraabdominal sepsis due to initial fecal contamination or subsequent suture line failure will gravitate to the pelvis. If not, the drains can be readily removed. If pelvic abscess does occur, drainage will be available. The occasional instance of sacral osteomyelitis complicating this procedure is not a sufficient contraindication.

The most common complication associated with colon injury is wound infection.[48] For this reason, it is generally advocated that the skin and subcutaneous tissue be left open after closure of peritoneum and fascia.[43] Delayed primary closure of the more superficial layers of the abdomen can be accomplished on about the fifth day following the initial operative procedure. Otherwise, closure can be postponed until the wound appears healthy and the patient is generally well. As with delayed primary closure of debrided wounds elsewhere, when delayed primary closure of the abdomen is prolonged much beyond five days, closure becomes progressively more difficult, requiring undermining of skin and subcutaneous tissues and even more complicated plastic surgical procedures to accomplish reapproximation of the skin margins.

An additional point regarding contamination deserves emphasis. The exit wound of a bullet which has penetrated the intestine, should be considered contaminated. It should be debrided accordingly.[42]

The question often arises as to whether the exteriorized colon can be brought out through the gunshot wound of the abdominal wall. The answer is yes; the procedure has been used on a sufficient number of occasions* to justify its continued recommendation when appropriate. Enlargement of the penetrating abdominal injury to two fingerbreadths, which is the minimal size that will reliably accept a diverted colon, is sufficient debridement of the wound itself, and the presence of the colostomy sufficient drainage, to prevent an anticipated complication such as entrance/colostomy wound abscess.

There is an additional point regarding colonic wounds and their management. Despite the relative safety and security in carrying out a colostomy and predicting its success, the disadvantage particularly of a double-barreled colostomy is that definitive surgery to restore continuity of the colon will itself carry significant morbidity and mortality. Morbidity of 22% has been reported.[54] Thus, despite warnings to the contrary, one is justified in considering primary repair of injuries to the colon despite the complications discussed above.

The Great Vessels

Penetrating injuries to the great vessels of the abdomen and pelvis remain a challenging problem to the trauma surgeon. Such injuries can be divided into those associated with an intact, and those associated with a penetrated, peritoneum, particularly when veins are injured. When the bleeding remains extraperitoneal, it may be self-limiting due to tissue resistance. In gunshot wounds of the abdomen or pelvis, such is rarely the case. If arterial exsanguination appears imminent emergency left thoracotomy and aortic cross-clamping are indicated. The latter procedure can be carried out rapidly, relatively safely, and often effectively.

---

*Authors' experience.

Probably the most challenging injury facing the surgeon is that involving penetration of the aorta in the region of the celiac or superior mesenteric arteries. Unless flow through these vessels is promptly restored fatal visceral necrosis will result. Probably the best approach is a rapid extraperitoneal mobilization of the spleen and pancreas away from the left lateral abdominal wall, to expose the aorta and its branches high in the abdomen. If a viscus has been penetrated vascular prosthetic material (cloth) probably should not be used. Such vascular injuries can be repaired with either direct anastomosis or utilization of interposition autogenous saphenous vein grafts.

Traumatic injuries to the inferior vena cava continue to carry a high mortality rate,[55] despite many innovative techniques designed to bypass the injury, allowing more time and better visibility for safe repair. Thus, among patients with vena caval injuries admitted to major trauma centers, 44% to 53% succumb despite surgical intervention.[56,57] The mortality is especially high with suprarenal inferior vena caval injuries, as compared to infrarenal inferior vena caval injuries. This difference reflects greater ease of exposure with the latter. The inferior vena cava, as well as the abdominal aorta, can be cross-clamped with partially occluding vascular instruments to permit lateral suture technique, simplifying vascular reconstruction.

A technique which has found application in controlling intraabdominal hemorrhage stems from the principle described by Crile at the turn of the century now known as the G-suit or MAST (Medical Anti-Shock Trousers). This apparatus encompasses the patient's body from the costal margin to the toes. It can be inflated safely to a pressure of 30 cm of saline for up to 24 hours.[58] Insertion of a Foley catheter is a prerequisite. Ventilatory assistance may also be required. While not recommended for control of suspected intraabdominal arterial hemorrhage, the G-suit has found successful application postoperatively when problems with blood coagulation such as disseminated intravascular coagulopathy have occurred.[58] The MAST has found additional application to hemorrhage attending pelvic and femoral fractures.

An additional challenging problem facing the trauma surgeon is the gunshot wound to the pelvis which may generate secondary missiles of bone and cause multiple injuries to branches of the pelvic venous plexuses (internal iliac, prostatic, etc.).[59] A mortality of 50% has been reported.[59] Since gunshot wounds are most frequently seen in males, the surgeon is usually faced with a relatively more difficult surgical exposure of the pelvis. Depending upon the availability of whole blood, exsanguination in the operating room is common. Attempts at suture ligation, cautery, clipping, clamping, and ligating are all made difficult by the rapidity with which the relatively small pelvic cavity fills with blood, despite the employment of multiple suction units. Packing is an alternative. However, the pack must be removed, and bleeding frequently recurs, as vigorously as at the time of the initial injury. Ligation of major vessels (hypogastric arteries) rarely helps because of the extensive collateral circulation in the pelvis. Similarly, arterial embolization utilizing radiographic techniques from above and below and such substances as autogenous blood clots, powdered Gelfoam, sodium morrhuate, or glass beads, may not provide a satisfactory solution to the problem despite an occasional report to the contrary. The MAST unit, although more applicable to pelvic fractures in which the peritoneum has not been opened, may play a role in the postoperative management of this problem[58] once bleeding has been temporarily controlled with appropriate absorbable packing material such as Gelfoam and Surgisel. Clearly, this remains a vexing and controversial problem for the surgeon and one which, at the present time, awaits some innovative approach if attendant morbidity and mortality are to be reduced.[60]

A variety of techniques for abdominal closure is available. Perhaps the simplest is the use of #28-gauge stainless steel wire in figure-of-eight fashion through the linea alba. In this technique, no attempt is made to close the peritoneum. Depending upon the degree of intra-abdominal contamination, the skin margins can be left open and closed secondarily approximately five days later. Instillation of antibiotic solution into the peritoneal cavity at the time of closure has been advocated by some, but evidence for its effectiveness is not compelling. The use of peritoneal irrigation with large quantities of saline has been advocated by many to reduce the degree of intraabdominal contamination, particularly if there has been significant soilage following injury to hollow viscera. The advantages that presumably result from such dilution may be outweighed by the dissemination of the contaminant throughout the peritoneal cavity, particularly into the pelvis and under the diaphragm.

SUMMARY

We believe that all gunshot wounds of the abdomen should be treated with exploratory laparotomy. A midline abdominal incision is preferable. If significant intraabdominal contamination exists, closure of the linea alba and peritoneum still can be accomplished safely; delayed primary closure of skin and subcutaneous tissue should await the fifth postoperative day. Preoperative evaluation should include radiograms of the chest and pelvis in anterior-posterior and lateral positions to evaluate potential thoracic or pelvic injury from the abdominal gunshot.

Injuries to small bowel are most common and are treated with simple closure or resection, as are those to the stomach. Injuries to the spleen are treated with splenectomy. The gallbladder is similarly

managed. Injuries to the liver are treated with drainage, suture ligation, or drainage and resection, depending upon the extent of the
damage. The Pringle maneuver is helpful in temporarily controlling
bleeding from the injured liver.

Damage to the pancreas and duodenum is treated in a variety of
ways depending upon the extent of injury, the degree of peritoneal
contamination, and the interval between injury and therapy. The
techniques of repair range from simple resection, closure or drainage,
to radical pancreaticoduodenectomy (Whipple procedure).

Injuries to the colon are similarly assessed and therapy ranges
from simple closure, most applicable to right colonic injuries, to
diverting colostomy, most applicable to left colonic injuries. The safest
treatment of either colonic injury is resection and double-barreled colostomy with a skin bridge between. In such cases, however, subsequent restoration of colonic function (anastomosis) will be a more formidable procedure than those associated with alternative primary
reparative techniques. Blood on the rectal examining finger implies
rectal injury and indicates diverting sigmoid colostomy, even if proctosigmoidoscopy and exploratory laparotomy prove negative. In fact,
we believe coccygectomy and prophylactic pelvic drainage are indicated in these circumstances together with irrigation of the rectum
from the sigmoidal and anal sides of the suspected injury. These
procedures are directed against anticipated pelvic abscess.

Major vascular injuries within the abdomen are problematic; if
arterial, primary repair with whatever technique available is required.
Aortic cross-clamping through a left thoracotomy will help control
blood loss. Mobilization of the spleen and left colon via dissection of
the left retroperitoneum facilitates exposure of the proximal portion
of the abdominal aorta and its branches. This maneuver can be
accomplished within a few minutes. Lateral suture is applicable to
relatively small and isolated injuries to the aorta or its major branches.
More extensive injury requires primary anastomosis. Injuries to major
veins are similarly treated. The exception is when the posterior
peritoneum is intact, in which case observation may be preferred.

Gunshot wounds of the pelvis pose a formidable problem in that
peritoneal penetration is implied, and secondary missiles are common.
Here, a variety of techniques to control hemorrhage is available to the
trauma surgeon, but as always, their number attests to the frustration
attending each. External compression with the G-suit or MAST may
prove the desired alternative, both pre- and postoperatively, to direct
surgical correction through ligation or repair.

153

REFERENCES

1. Maughon, J.S. An inquiry into the nature of wounds resulting in killed in action in Vietnam. *Milit Med.* 135:8–13, 1970.
2. *Emergency War Surgery.* U.S. Armed Forces Issue of NATO Handbook. Prepared for use by the Medical Services of NATO Nations. Washington, D.C.: U.S. Government Printing Office, 1958, p. 18.
3. Lowe, R.J., Saletta, J.D., Read, D.R. et al. Should laparotomy be mandatory or selective in gunshot wounds of the abdomen? *J Trauma.* 17:903–907, 1977.
4. Lucas, C.E. The role of peritoneal lavage for penetrating abdominal wounds. Editorial. *J Trauma.* 17:649–650, 1977.
5. Thal, E.R. Evaluation of peritoneal lavage and local exploration in lower chest and abdominal stab wounds. *J Trauma.* 17:642–648, 1977.
6. Topilow, A.A., and Steinhoff, N.G. Splenic pseudocyst: a late complication of trauma. *J Trauma.* 15:260–263, 1975.
7. Bell, R.P. Splenic cysts with report of a case of a large unilocular cyst of rapid growth. *Ann Surg.* 137:781–786, 1953.
8. Clark, O.H., Lim, R.C., and Margaretten, W. Spontaneous delayed splenic rupture: Case report of a five-year interval between trauma and diagnosis. *J Trauma.* 15:245–249, 1975.
9. Ballinger, W.F., Erslen, A.J. Splenectomy indications, technique, and complications. *Curr Probl Surg.* February 1965, pp. 1–51.
10. Olsen, W.R. and Polley, T.Z. A second look at delayed splenic rupture. *Arch Surg.* 112:422–425, 1977.
11. Lowenfels, A.B. Kehr's sign—A neglected aid in rupture of the spleen. *New Engl J Med.* 274:1019, 1966.
12. Polin, S.G. Walklett, W.D., and Sayler, O.L. Arteriography as an adjunct to the diagnosis of splenic injury. *Surgery* 67:313–318, 1970.
13. O'Mara, R.E., Hall, R.C., and Dombroski, D.L. Scintiscanning in the diagnosis of rupture of the spleen. *Surg Gynecol Obstet.* 131:1077–1084, 1970.
14. McLelland, R.N., Jones, R.C., Shires, G.T. et al. Trauma to the abdomen. Edited by G.T. Shires. In *Care of the Trauma Patient.* New York: McGraw-Hill Book Co., 1966, pp. 397–400.
15. Sizer, J.S., Wayne, E.R., and Frederick, P.L. Delayed rupture of the spleen: review of the literature and report of six cases. *Arch Surg.* 92:362–366, 1966.
16. Lieberman, R.C., and Welch, C.S. A study of 248 instances of traumatic rupture of the spleen. *Surg Gynecol Obstet.* 127:961–965, 1968.
17. Pringle, J.H. Notes on arrest of hepatic hemorrhage. *Ann Surg.* 48:541, 1908.
18. Mays, E.T., Hepatic trauma. *Curr Probl Surg.* 13:1–73, 1976.
19. Levin, A., Gover, P., and Nance, F.C. Surgical restraint in the management of hepatic injury: a review of Charity Hospital experience *J Trauma.* 18:399–404, 1978.
20. DeFore, W.W. Mattox, K.L., Jordan, G.L. et al. Management of 1590 consecutive cases of liver trauma. *Arch Surg.* 111:493–497, 1976.
21. Trunkey, D.D., Shires, G.T., and McClelland, R. Management of liver trauma in 811 consecutive patients. *Ann Surg.* 179:722–728, 1974.

22. Nance, F.C., Wennar, M.H., Johnson, L.W. et al. Surgical judgment in the management of penetrating wounds of the abdomen: experience with 2212 patients. *Ann Surg.* 179:639–646, 1974.

23. Davis, J.J., Cohn, I., and Nance, F.C. Diagnosis and management of blunt abdominal trauma. *Ann Surg.* 183:672–678, 1976.

24. Lucas, C.E., and Ledgerwood, A.M. Prospective evaluation of hemostatic techniques for liver injuries. *J Trauma.* 16:442–451, 1976.

25. Drezner, A.D., and Foster, J.H. Decreasing morbidity after liver trauma. *Am J Surg.* 129:483–489, 1975.

26. Mercadier, M.P., Clot, J.P., and Cady, J.P. Right hepatectomy in the treatment of liver trauma. *Am J Surg.* 124:353–358, 1972.

27. Jona, J.Z. Ligation of the main hepatic artery for exsanguinating liver laceration in an adolescent. *J Trauma.* 18:225–226, 1978.

28. Schrock, T., Blaisdell, F.W., and Mathewson, C. Management of blunt trauma to the liver and hepatic veins. *Arch Surg.* 96:698–704, 1968.

29. Perry, J.F. Blunt and penetrating abdominal injuries. Edited by M.M. Ravitch. In *Current Problems in Surgery.* Chicago: Yearbook Medical Publishers, May, 1970, pp. 19–31.

30. Sandblom, P. Hemorrhage into the biliary tract following trauma: "traumatic hemobilia." *Surgery* 24:571–586, 1948.

31. Graham, J.M., Mattox, K.L., and Beall, A.C., Portal venous system injuries. *J Trauma.* 18:419–422, 1978.

32. Kelly, G., Norton, L., Moore, G. et al. The continuing challenge of duodenal injuries. *J Trauma.* 18:160–165, 1978.

33. Corley, R.D., Norcross, W.J., and Shoemaker, W.C. Traumatic injuries to the duodenum: a report of 98 patients. *Ann Surg.* 181:92–98, 1975.

34. Morton, J.R., and Jordan, G.L. Traumatic duodenal injuries: review of 131 cases. *J Trauma.* 8:127–139, 1968.

35. Smith, A.D., Woolverton, W.C., Weichert, R.F. et al. Operative management of pancreatic and duodenal injuries. *J Trauma.* 11:570–576, 1971.

36. Berne, C.J., Donovan, A.J., White, E.J. et al. Duodenal "diverticulization" for duodenal and pancreatic injury. *Am J Surg.* 127:503–507, 1974.

37. Anderson, C.B., Weisz, D., Rodger, M.R. et al. Combined pancreaticoduodenal trauma. *Am J Surg.* 125:530–534, 1973.

38. Wolff, L.H., and Giddings, W.P. Penetrating wounds of the stomach, duodenum, and small intestine. *Surg Clin North Am.* 38:1605–1618, 1958.

39. Brawley, R.K., Cameron, J.L., and Zuidema, G.D. Severe upper abdominal injuries treated by pancreaticoduodenectomy. *Surg Gynecol Obstet.* 126:516–522, 1968.

40. McInnis, W.D., Aust, J.B., Cruz, A.B. et al. Traumatic injuries of the duodenum: a comparison of 1° closure and the jejunal patch. *J Trauma.* 15:847–853, 1975.

41. Lucas, C.E., and Ledgerwood, A.M. Factors influencing outcome after blunt duodenal injury. *J Trauma.* 15:839–846, 1975.

42. Josen, A.S. Ferrer, J.M. Forde, K.A. et al. Primary closure of civilian colorectal wounds. *Ann Surg.* 176:782–786, 1972.

43. Steele, M., and Blaisdell, F.W. Treatment of colon injuries. *J Trauma.* 17:557–562, 1977.

44. Haynes, C.D., Gunn, C.H., and Martin, J.D. Colon injuries. *Arch Surg.* 96:944–948, 1968.

45. Mason, J.M. Surgery of the colon in the forward battle area. *Surgery* 18:534–541, 1945.

46. Elkin, D.C., and Ward, W.C. Gunshot wounds of the abdomen: a survey of 238 cases. *Ann Surg.* 118:780–787, 1943.

47. LoCicero, J., Tajima, T., and Drapanas, T. A half-century of experience in the management of colon injuries: changing concepts. *J Trauma.* 15:575–581, 1975.

48. Mulherin, J.L., and Sawyers, J.L. Evaluation of three methods for managing penetrating colon injuries. *J Trauma.* 15:580–587, 1975.

49. Schrock, T.R., and Christensen, N. Management of perforating injuries of the colon. *Surg Gynecol Obstet.* 135:65–68, 1972.

50. Matolo, N.M., and Wolfman, E.F. Primary repair of colonic injuries: a clinical evaluation. *J Trauma.* 17:554–556, 1977.

51. Chilimindris, C., Boyd, D.R., Carlson, L.E. et al. A critical review of management of right colon injuries. *J Trauma.* 11:651–660, 1971.

52. Freeark, R.J. The injured colon. Editorial. *J Trauma.* 17:563–564, 1977.

53. Kirkpatrick, J.R., and Rajpal, S.G. The management of penetrating wounds of the colon. *Surg Gynecol Obstet.* 137:484–486, 1973.

54. Matolo, N.M., Cohen, S.E., Wolfman, E.F. Experimental evaluation of primary repair of colonic injuries. *Arch Surg.* 111:78–80, 1976.

55. Cheek, R.C., Pope, J.C., Smith, H.F., et al. Diagnosis and management of major vascular injuries: a review of 200 operative cases. *Am Surg.* 41:755–760, 1975.

56. Allen, R.E., and Blaisdell, F.W. Injuries to the inferior vena cava. *Surg Clin North Am.* 52:699–710, 1972.

57. Turpin, I., State, D., and Schwartz, A. Injuries to the inferior vena cava and their management. *Am J Surg.* 134:25–32, 1977.

58. Burdick, J.F., Warshaw, A.L., and Abbott, W.M. External counter-pressure to control postoperative intra-abdominal hemorrhage. *Am J Surg.* 129:369–373, 1975.

59. Rothenberger, D., Velasco, R., Strate, R., et al. Open pelvic fracture: a lethal injury. *J Trauma.* 18:184–187, 1978.

60. Greico, J.G., and Perry, J.F. Retroperitoneal hematoma following trauma: Its significance. *J Trauma.* (In press) Presented at the 39th Annual Meeting of the American Association for the Surgery of Trauma. Chicago, September 13–15, 1979.

8 The Genitourinary Tract

If the kidney or bladder is penetrated, the escape of urine into the abdomen is almost a certain cause of fatal result.*

Up to 1931 only seven such cases (ureteral wounds induced by firearms) had been reported in the medical literature (Le Compte) and even in wartime gunshot injuries to the ureter appear to be very rare.†

We are aware of no report of a penetrating wound of the abdomen, during pregnancy, not involving the uterus.‡

Gunshot wounds of the genitourinary tract nearly always result in gross hematuria (Figures 8-1 through 8-17). Thus, transurethral catheterization of the bladder is mandatory when there is any possibility that the wound may have involved the genitourinary tract. The urine is almost invariably bright red, in part because positive intraluminal pressure in the genitourinary tract opposes any significant venous bleeding into the tract itself.

*Longmore, T. *Gunshot Wounds.* Philadelphia: J.B. Lippincott Co., 1863.
†Lowsley, O.S., and Kirwin, T.J. *Clinical Urology,* ed 2, vol 3. Baltimore: Williams & Wilkins Co., 1944.
‡Dyer, I., and Barclay, D. Accidental trauma complicating pregnancy and delivery. *Am J Obstet Gynecol.* 83:907, 1962.

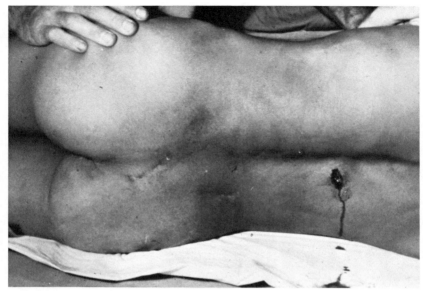

Figure 8-1 A 41-year-old farmer sustained this 82-mm mortar fragment wound of his back. (Figures 8-1 through 8-7 courtesy U.S. Army–Vietnam Surgical Trauma Collection, Armed Forces Institute of Pathology, Washington, D.C.)

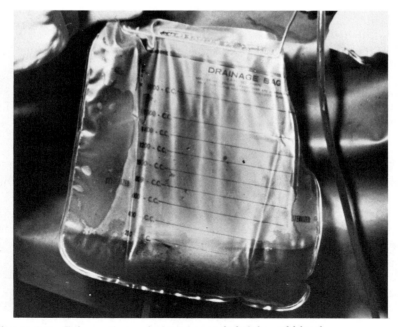

Figure 8-2 Foley catheter drainage reveals bright-red blood.

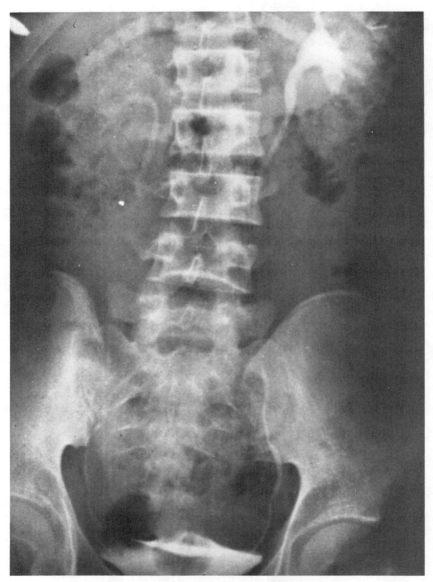

Figure 8-3 Intravenous pyelography reveals delayed function on the right and a metallic foreign body located in the right upper abdominal quadrant. The apparent metallic foreign body in the middle third of the right ureter is an artifact.

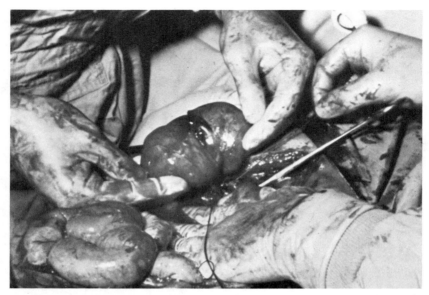

Figure 8-4   At surgery, the right kidney exhibits a lateral cortical defect and a dusky upper pole. Nephrectomy was elected as the procedure of choice.

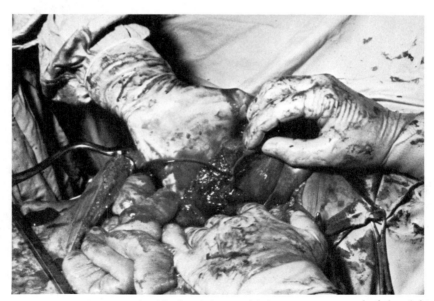

Figure 8-5   Associated with the right renal injury was a wound of the right lobe of the liver. The jet of blood seen is in obvious need of hemostatic control, and this was accomplished with suture ligation following debridement.

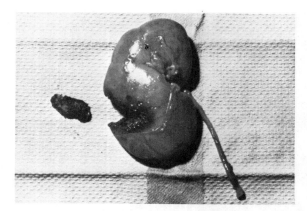

Figure 8-6 The resected right kidney along with the wounding agent are exhibited. A partial nephrectomy would have been an alternative possibility and might have preserved at least 50% of unilateral renal function. This procedure, although recommended by urologists for obvious reasons, was accomplished relatively infrequently during the Vietnam War due to the fact that there often existed significant numbers of associated injuries, and control of hemorrhage which attended the renal injury was singly best accomplished by nephrectomy as quickly as possible, so as to permit attention to the other areas of equally significant, or more important, trauma.

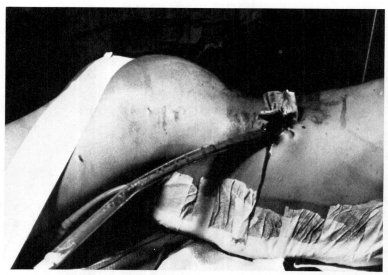

Figure 8-7 Dependent drainage with both sump tube and Penrose drains is indicated in the management of this type of injury. Both the renal bed and hepatic lobar suture repair are sources of blood accumulation, and in the case of the liver, bile accumulation as well. These fluids need egress via appropriately placed drains, but it must be remembered that the sump tube (semi-rigid), if left in place too long (greater than 48–72 hours), may lead to erosion through vital structures, especially hollow viscera, with attendant disastrous complications.

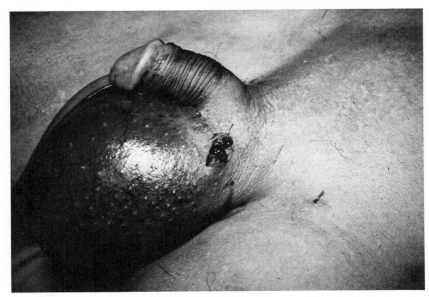

Figure 8-8 An M-16 gunshot wound of a 29-year-old male, has caused a scrotal hematoma.

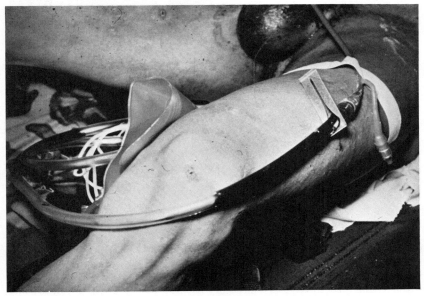

Figure 8-9 The Foley catheter bladder drainage is at first dark red.

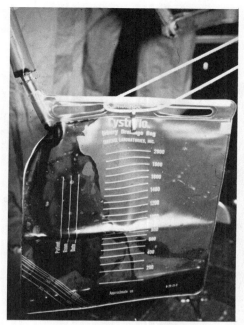

Figure 8-10 The Foley catheter drainage then becomes bright red.

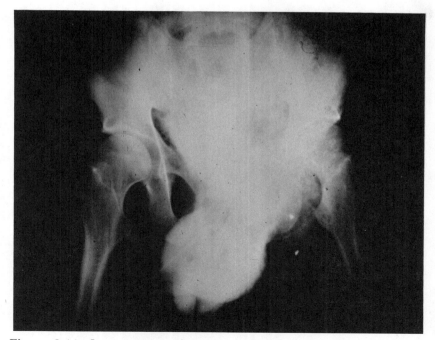

Figure 8-11 Intravenous pyelography is negative, but cystogram reveals extravasation into the peritoneal cavity and scrotum.

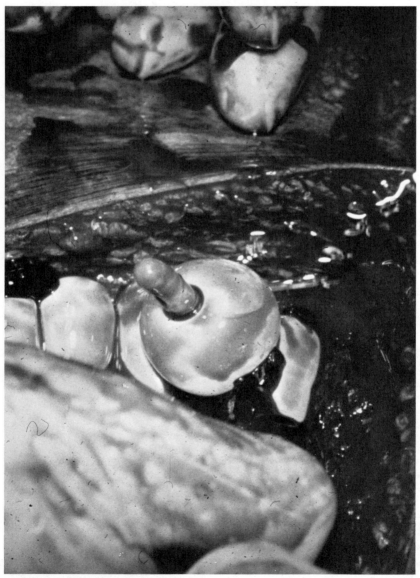

Figure 8-12 Abdominal exploration reveals the Foley catheter in the incision confirming the bladder defect.

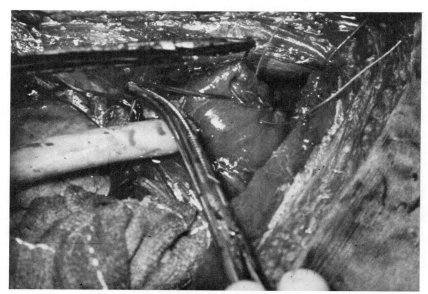

Figure 8-13 The bladder is repaired over a cystostomy tube and in layers with chromic catgut.

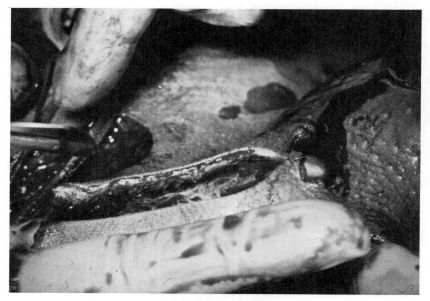

Figure 8-14 The scrotal contents are explored via an inguinal incision.

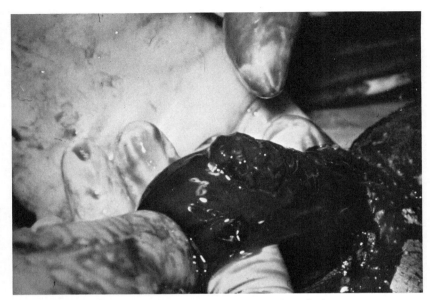

Figure 8-15   An injury to the spermatic cord is identified.

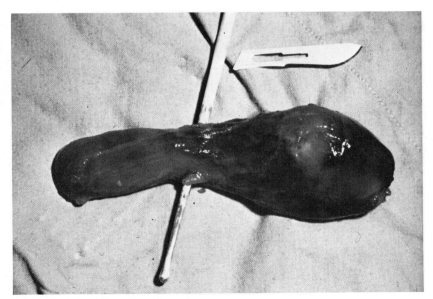

Figure 8-16   An inguinal orchiectomy is performed and the bullet probe reveals the through-and-through wound of the cord.

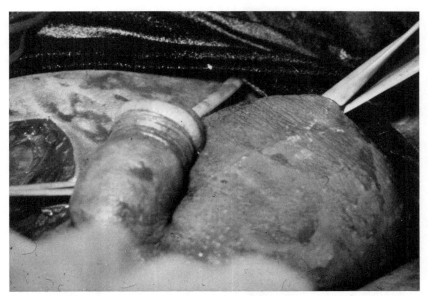

Figure 8-17   The scrotum is closed primarily, but a Penrose drain is inserted.

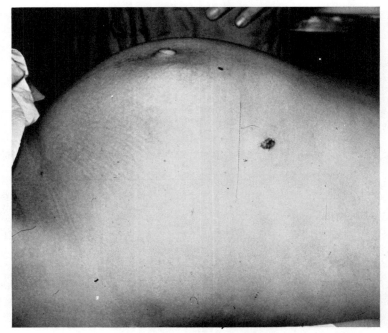

Figure 8-18   A female, age 23, was shot in the abdomen with an M-2 carbine. She is seven months pregnant and the fetus is viable.

168

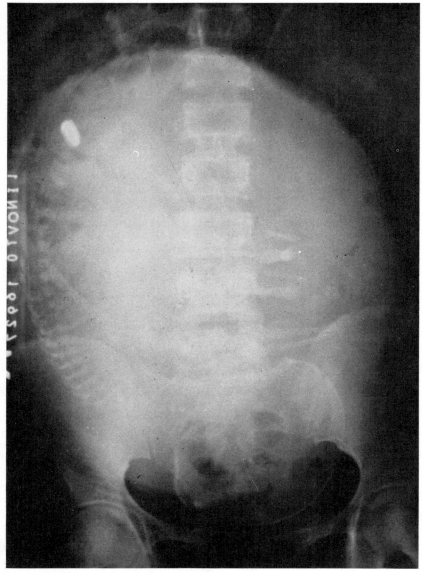

Figure 8-19 A-P and lateral radiograms of the abdomen reveal a fetal skeleton. . .

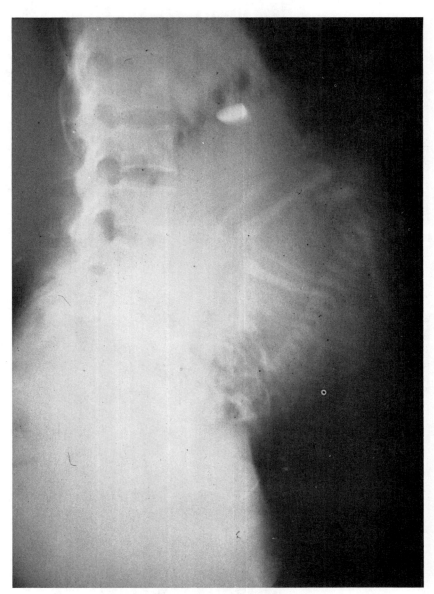

Figure 8-20 . . .and a bullet in the upper abdomen.

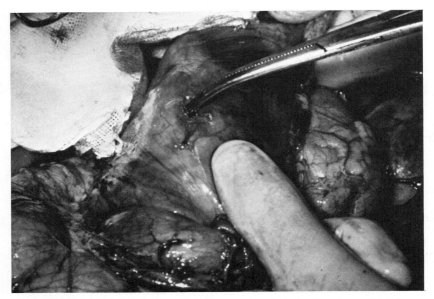

Figure 8-21 Exploratory laparotomy reveals a hole in the stomach and. . .

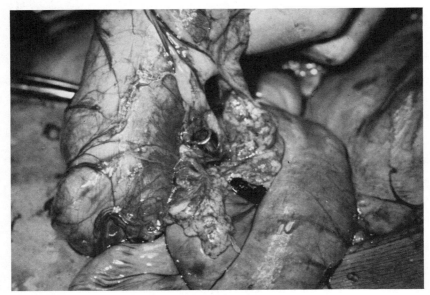

Figure 8-22 . . .a bullet in the lesser sac.

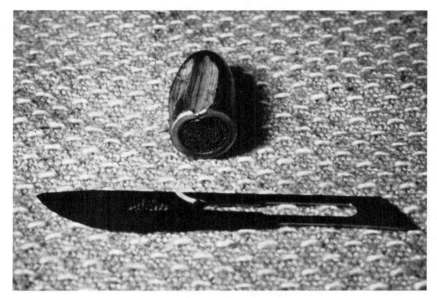

Figure 8-23 The bullet is removed and appears to have ricocheted before striking the patient.

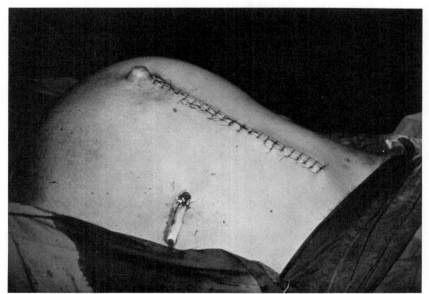

Figure 8-24 The abdomen is closed and a single Penrose drain brought out through the entrance wound. The patient survived and delivered a normal baby at term.

When gross hematuria is evident following wounding, transurethral catheterization is required for diagnostic, as well as therapeutic reasons. Intravenous pyelography is indicated and may reveal: (1) delayed or absent urine flow on one or both sides (Figure 8-3); (2) extravasation of contrast media from the kidney or the ureter; or (3) the existence or absence of the contralateral kidney. Since most penetrating injuries of the kidney are treated by nephrectomy, existence of the contralateral kidney is an important consideration. Intravenous pyelography is indicated in the absence of hematuria if the apparent path of the bullet approaches either ureter or kidney, since penetrating injury to the urinary tract occasionally is associated with normal urine. Cystoscopy is contraindicated in these circumstances, since distention of the bladder with clear fluid is an essential part of the diagnostic procedure and would be unsuccessful in the presence of an injury to the bladder.

If intravenous pyelography is negative, cystographic examination is the next step and may reveal injury to the bladder as the presumptive source of bleeding (Figure 8-11). In both males and females, bleeding from the urethral orifice suggests injury to the urethra, as does difficulty in passing a Foley catheter. To localize a urethral injury in the male, a urethrogram may be obtained by injecting contrast material directly into the urethra with a bulb syringe.

MANAGEMENT

The Kidney

Since gunshot injury is rarely restricted to the genitourinary tract, its operative management usually coincides with exploratory laparotomy and repair of additional injuries of other abdominal and pelvic structures. Injury to the right kidney by gunshot is often associated with injury to the right colon, duodenum, and right lobe of the liver (Figure 8-5); that to the left kidney is frequently accompanied by injury to the pancreas, spleen, and left colon. Because of these serious associated injuries, renal laceration is usually treated by nephrectomy (Figure 8-4). Such was the case in the Vietnam War. However, whenever safe and possible, the preservation of renal function by subtotal nephrectomy should be considered. The risk is postoperative hemorrhage and formation of a paraspinal abscess.

Emergency nephrectomy for trauma is readily accomplished through the standard midline abdominal incision regardless of whether the right or left side is involved. The distal stump of the ureter should be ligated. Because of the blunt dissection required, the probable extravasation of urine, and associated injury to the liver or pancreas, the renal bed should be drained with several Penrose tubes for the first day or two postoperatively. A sump tube should be positioned, but not left in place for more than 72 hours, since the chance of its erosion into viscera or major vessels increases with time (Figure 8-7). As in partial hepatectomy, partial nephrectomy is accomplished with the technique of finger fracture, ligating major branches of the renal artery and veins, as well as major calyces. In all genitourinary tract surgery, absorbable suture material is preferred (Figure 8-13), except in the ligation of major blood vessels.

The Ureter

Occasionally, the ureter is the only viscus injured in a gunshot wound of the abdomen and pelvis. It is best treated by drainage of the injured region, primary repair over a ureteral catheter, and exteriorization of the catheter through a separate stab wound distal to the repair. If the ureter is only partially divided, drainage alone may be all that is necessary, as the experience with ureterolithotomy shows. When the ureter is drained, the chance of luminal obstruction by scar formation is unlikely, unless the injury is circumferential. Injury to the distal third of the ureter is probably best treated with ureteral reimplantation. When a long segment of ureter is destroyed, the kidney can sometimes be autotransplanted to the pelvis.

The Bladder

Injury to the bladder is readily apparent when the Foley catheter is visualized upon opening the abdominal cavity (Figure 8-12). Injuries of the dome of the bladder are easily managed with closure of the bladder wall in two layers using either continuous or interrupted absorbable suture material. A suprapubic cystostomy tube is advisable to facilitate bladder drainage following this repair and to enable early mobilization of the urethral catheter which, in the case of males, can cause an ascending infection culminating in epididymitis (Figure 8-13). The suprapubic cystostomy tube is usually a Malecot or mushroom catheter which can be brought out through the abdominal incision. Following bladder repair, the prevesical space should be drained with a single Penrose tube. Injuries to the bladder neck are more challenging and at the time of surgery, frequently require catheterization of both ureteral orifices in order to prevent their suture ligation during bladder reconstruction. Where question arises, operative use of intravenous methylene blue may help identify defects in the ureters or their orifices within the bladder. An omental pedicle graft may find application to repairing larger defects.[1]

The Urethra

Injury to the urethra may require passage of catheters from proximal and distal orifices in order to establish communication between urethral orifice and bladder neck. This is necessary for successful restoration of epithelial continuity along the injured urethra. Under these circumstances, the external genitalia should be included in the operative field. Urethral injury indicates cystostomy in the manner previously described, as well as urethral catheter splinting and drainage. Stricture is a probable late complication which should be anticipated, and about which the patient should be made cognizant.

The Male Genitalia

The external genitalia in the male constitute one of the four anatomical areas (head, neck, chest, external genitalia) where even high-velocity gunshot wounds are successfully treated with debridement and primary closure, as opposed to delayed primary closure appropriate to the management of such wounds elsewhere. That is because primary closure is usually necessary to arrest hemorrhage. Experience shows that such practice is well tolerated. Injury to the scrotal contents is usually treated with inguinal orchiectomy and primary closure of the scrotum. Dependent Penrose drainage is indicated (Figures 8-14–8-17). Bilateral testicular injury is relatively uncommon. When it does occur, tissue salvage and ultimate partial preservation of endocrine, as well as sexual function, indicate subtotal resection wherever possible. The same is true of penetrating injury of the abdomen which involves one or more ovaries, although this is an unusually rare injury.

The Gravid Uterus

Gunshot wounds of the patient with a gravid uterus are not uncommon, either during wartime, or in civilian life, and their management in general pertains to the viability of the fetus in terms of its gestational period (Figures 8-18–8-24). A number of physiologic considerations should be kept in mind during evaluation of potential injury to the pregnant patient. Physiologic hypervolemia accompanies pregnancy, and it has been estimated that circulating blood volume has increased by 50% at the 30th to 34th week of pregnancy.[2] Thus, for the trauma surgeon attending a patient with an intrauterine pregnancy who has sustained a gunshot wound of the abdomen or pelvis, the physiologic hypervolemia of pregnancy is a two-edged sword; that is, the hypervolemia protects the mother in terms of permitting her to tolerate considerably larger volumes of blood loss than her nonpregnant counterpart, but at the same time, threatens the fetus who experiences significant threat from hypoxemia with any reduction in maternal blood volume.

In addition, during pregnancy central venous pressure falls progressively, and at term, is approximately one-third of its usual level.[3] For obvious reasons, during initial evaluation of gunshot wounds of the abdomen, peritoneal lavage should be employed with caution. The risk of injury to the intestine and uterus by lavage is considerable, and the value of lavage of the compartmentalized peritoneal cavity is reduced in the pregnant patient. The physiologic leukocytosis of as much as 50% above normal accompanying pregnancy is another phenomenon which should be kept in mind in the management of gunshot wounds in the pregnant patient.[4] Bilateral hydronephrosis and hydroureter of pregnancy must also be considered in interpreting pyelograms in the wounded patient.[2]

When laparotomy is necessary, it is advisable to have an obstetrician attend the procedure and a pediatrician available. Some believe that cesarean section is usually indicated only when: (1) surgical access to other wounded structures is impeded; (2) if there is hemorrhage from, or injury to, fetus, placenta, or umbilical cord; or (3) there is impending infection.[2] Others develop reasons for more liberal resort to cesarean section in patients with abdominal or pelvic gunshot wounds. They believe the postoperative course following repair of the wound is compromised by the risk of labor and vaginal delivery, given the existence of a recent large abdominal incision. They also point out the risk of postoperative pulmonary complications from increased intraabdominal pressure and decreased diaphragmatic excursion.[5]

The anesthetic of choice is intravenous sodium pentothal, nitrous oxide, and oxygen along with succinylcholine. The last does not cross the placental barrier and will not interfere with neonatal respiratory movements, as might curare.[5]

Unidentified constituents of amniotic fluid have been reported to be a source of disseminated intravascular coagulation ("amniotic fluid embolism").[6] This consideration has led some to advocate the need for early and aggressive evacuation of the uterus and embryo.[6] The counterargument poses the probability that amniotic fluid embolism is extremely rare and is usually the result of a retained dead fetus and accompanying syndrome.[7]

Damage by gunshot wounds to pelvic structures comprising the birth canal is a significant consideration.[8] Approximately 50% of women who sustain pelvic fractures prior to or during pregnancy have normal vaginal deliveries. Twenty-five precent require cesarean section because of cephalopelvic disproportion consequent to the pelvic injury. In 25%, the fetus is lost as a result of the pelvic fracture. As might be expected, the fetal loss is higher when fracture occurs during pregnancy. In the management of gunshot wounds of the pelvis in women, there need be concern for potential complications of future pregnancies consequent to the gunshot wound.

In decisions regarding continuing or terminating pregnancy in the face of gunshot wounds, the desires and ethical convictions of the wounded patient must be given prominent consideration.

SUMMARY

In summary, gross hematuria almost invariably accompanies penetrating injury of the genitourinary tract. Catheterization is required for the prompt recognition of hematuria. Intravenous pyelography, cystography, or urethrography will identify the location of the injury. Although nephrectomy for renal injury may be necessary, consideration should be given to preserving renal function by partial nephrectomy. Renal or ureteral injuries require drainage. Injuries to the bladder should be closed primarily over a suprapubic cystostomy tube utilizing a two-layer anastomosis with absorbable suture material. Wounds of the external genitalia can be debrided and closed primarily. Of special concern are abdominal and pelvic gunshot wounds in pregnancy, wherein the decision to terminate pregnancy involves consideration of access to and repair of other wounded structures, the recovery of the wounded mother, access to the wounded fetus, and the desires and ethical considerations of the mother.

REFERENCES

1. Murphy, J.J., Malloy, T.R., and Wein, A.J. The omental pedicle as an aid in genitourinary reconstructive procedures. *J Trauma.* (In press) Presented at the 39th Annual Meeting of the American Association for the Surgery of Trauma. Chicago, September 13–15, 1979.

2. Buchsbaum, H.J. Diagnosis and management of abdominal gunshot wounds during pregnancy. *J Trauma.* 15:425–430, 1975.

3. Colditz, R.B., and Josey, W.E. Central venous pressure in supine position during normal pregnancy: comparative determinations during first, second, and third trimesters. *Obstet Gynecol.* 36:769–772, 1970.

4. Mitchell, G.W., McRipley, R.J., Selvaraj, R.J. et al. The role of the phagocyte in host-parasite interactions. IV. The phagocytic activity of leukocytes in pregnancy and its relationship to urinary tract infections. *Am J Obstet Gynecol.* 96:687–697, 1966.

5. Wright, J.K., McNamara, J.J., and Brief, D.K. The management of acute penetrating abdominal trauma complicating term pregnancy. *J Trauma.* 11:87–89, 1971.

6. Sheldon, G.F. Discussion of Buchsbaum, H.J., "Diagnosis and management of abdominal gunshot wounds during pregnancy." 34th Annual Session of the American Association for the Surgery of Trauma. Hot Springs, Va., October 1974.

7. Buchsbaum, H.J. Closing Summary. 34th Annual Session of the American Association for the Surgery of Trauma, Hot Springs, Va., October 1974.

8. Speer, D.P., and Peltier, L.F. Pelvic fractures and pregnancy. *J Trauma.* 12:474–480, 1972.

9 The Extremities

If the femoral artery and vein have been lacerated, any attempt to preserve the limb will certainly prove fatal.*

The severity of gunshot wounds of extremities depends upon the involvement of bone, great vessels, and nerves, not on the extent of skin and muscle damage. Thus, a through-and-through gunshot wound of the calf which does not strike bone or major neurovascular structures may, in fact, heal uneventfully without surgical intervention. By contrast, a high-velocity missile wound, apparently limited to skin and muscle, may include severe cavitational damage to bone, vessels, and nerves relatively remote from the missile tract. Therefore, every effort should be made to assess the ballistics of the wound. Recall that the M-16 round is of about the same caliber and weight, but has four times the velocity of that fired by a 22-caliber handgun and hits with 25 times the kinetic energy. The superficial appearance of the wound may not

---

*Longmore, T. *Gunshot Wounds.* Philadelphia: J.B. Lippincott Co., 1863.

be apparently different in the two cases. However, a fatality or an amputation may hinge upon this distinction. At operation, the difference is readily apparent. The wound inflicted by the handgun may require little or no surgical therapy. That induced by the M-16 requires radical debridement (Figures 9-1–9-17).

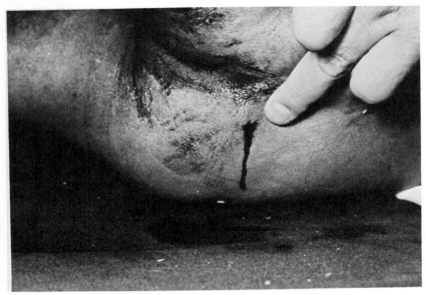

Figure 9-1 Small entrance wound in right buttock from M-16 rifle round fired from 150 m. Victim is a 31-year-old male.

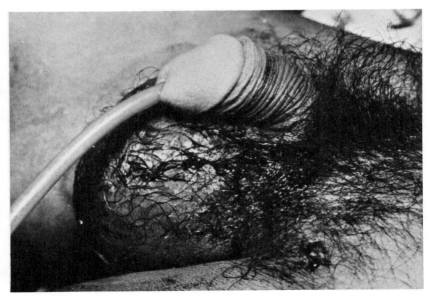

Figure 9-2 Small exit wound in the left groin is the only other skin injury.

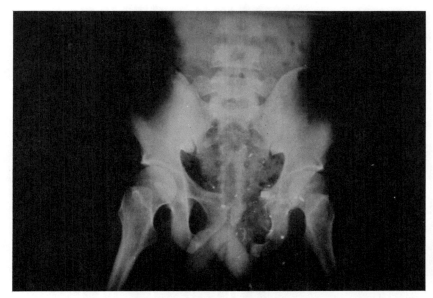

Figure 9-3 Radiographic examination of the pelvis reveals multiple metallic foreign bodies and destruction of the left superior and inferior pubic rami. This radiogram would have been interpreted as "multiple fragment wounds" without the knowledge that there were only two skin breaks and, in fact, that the causative weapon was an M-16. Tumbling and disintegration on impact are characteristic of this high-velocity missile, particularly if bone is in its path.

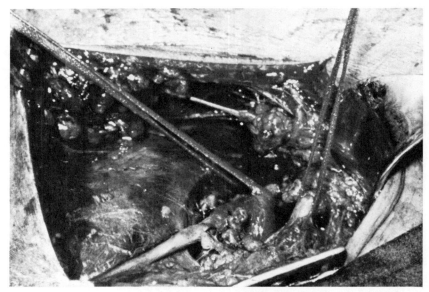

Figure 9-4 Because of the proximity of the only exit wound to the left femoral vessels, the latter underwent surgical exploration, which proved negative. Umbilical tapes surround the common femoral artery and vein.

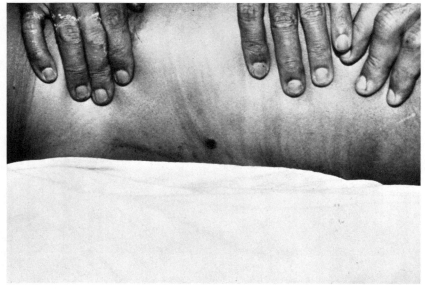

Figure 9-5 A 36-year-old male was injured by two M-16 rifle rounds fired from a distance of 30 m. One round entered his right flank.

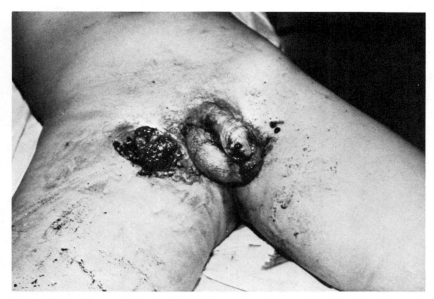

Figure 9-6 The round exited his right groin and caused perineal ecchymosis and injury to the external genitalia.

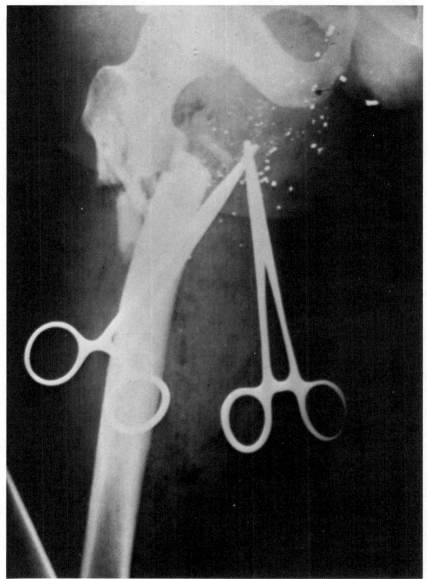

Figure 9-7 Radiographically, there is a comminuted, displaced fracture of the proximal right femur. Multiple metallic densities are characteristic of M-16 rifle rounds. The clamps are controlling arterial hemorrhage. They are not vascular clamps, unfortunately.

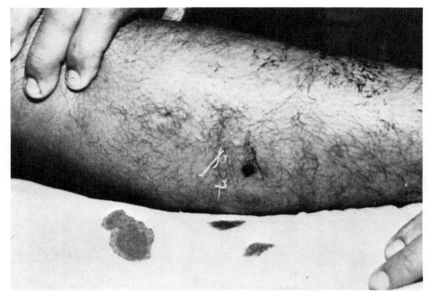

Figure 9-8 The second round struck the patient's right leg laterally.

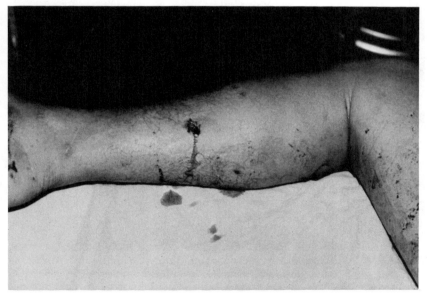

Figure 9-9 The round exited medially and did not encounter bone.

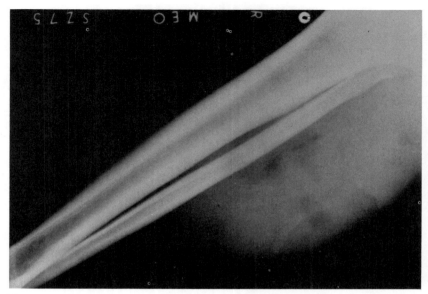

Figure 9-10 Radiographic examination of the right leg reveals no fracture or foreign body.

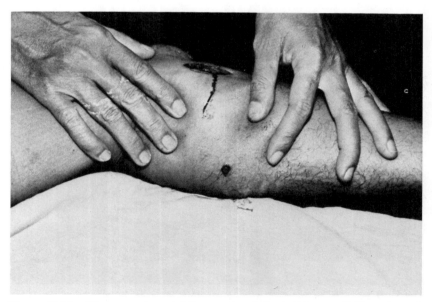

Figure 9-11 The second round then entered the left leg medially, where it struck bone.

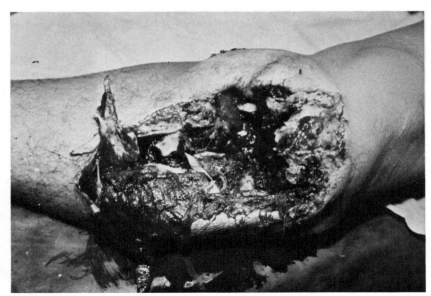

Figure 9-12 The wound of exit of the left leg exhibits the massive tissue destruction characteristic of M-16 gunshot wounds in which bone is struck by the bullet.

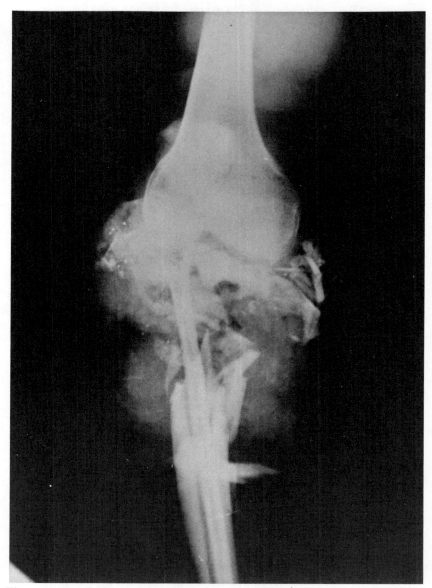

Figure 9-13 Radiographic examination of the left lower extremity verifies the clinically suspected destruction of the knee joint.

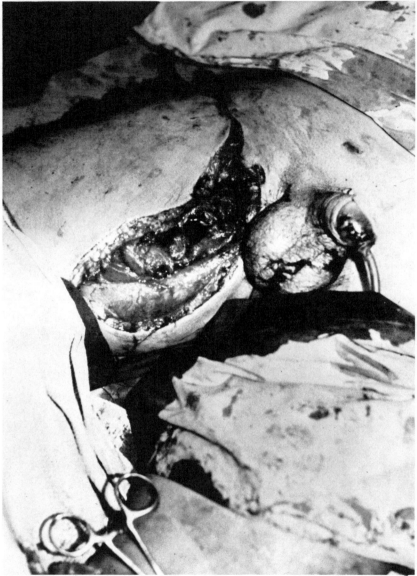

Figure 9-14 The first wound has been debrided. The femoral vessels were explored, found intact, and the wound closed primarily along its proximal and lateral extent. A branch of the profunda femoral artery, clamped during resuscitation, was ligated. The external genitalia have been debrided and closed primarily.

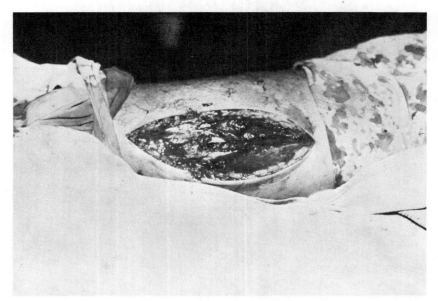

Figure 9-15 The extent of debridement necessary on the relatively less-injured right leg due to the extensive tissue destruction by the M-16 round.

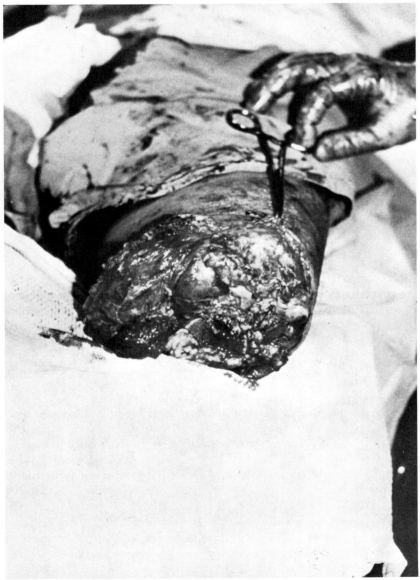

Figure 9-16 Guillotine amputation is the only treatment possible for the left lower extremity.

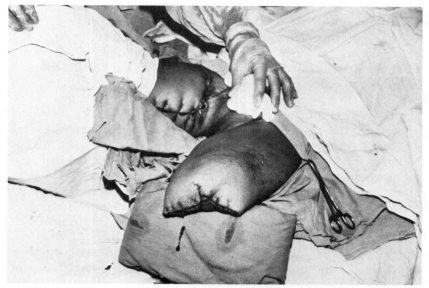

Figure 9-17 Delayed primary closure is carried out five days later. No attempt is made at cosmetic reconstruction of these wounds other than reapproximation of the skin margins.

A precise inquiry as to the wounding agent and pertinent examination precedes diagnostic tests and planned surgical intervention. Having ascertained the adequacy of respiration and circulation, attention must then be directed to minimizing additional damage to artery, vein, nerve, or bone.

DIAGNOSIS

Assuming that external hemorrhage has been controlled, the next immediate concern is the integrity of bony parts. Too often, the obvious injury to soft parts distracts the surgeon from the equally important, and more immediate, concern for long-bone fracture. With long-bone fracture comes the danger that the fracture may be made worse by movement of the extremity and nerves or blood vessels injured. The part must be inspected for angulation, disparity in length, and visible bony fragments. Injury to soft tissue alone may not be painful; pain suggests a fracture. Tenderness over bone, often exquisite, suggests fracture or subperiosteal contusion, whereas soft tissue is frequently painless immediately after penetrating injury. False or painful motion, as well as crepitation (palpable or audible gritting of fragments of bone), also indicates the likelihood of fracture. If fracture is probable, the extremity should be splinted immediately, as in the case of blunt trauma.

The next immediate concern is the presence or development of a hematoma, or of a more occult vascular injury. From an estimate of the extent of cavitation along the path of the missile and bearing in mind that complete occlusion of the major artery at the proximal end of a limb may exist without significant ischemia distally,[1] one must rigorously rule out major arterial injury. Sensation, motility, temperature, and color of the distal part of the extremity must be compared between the injured and uninjured limbs. The next step is assessment of distal arterial pulses by palpation, or more precisely, by measurement of Doppler systolic pressure. In the event that both paired limbs are injured, the Doppler systolic pressure is compared between an upper and lower extremity. These pressure measurements may indicate a compromise in arterial flow to the extremity unless core systemic arterial pressure is very low. In time, emergency rooms will be equipped with intraarterial pressure-monitoring devices which would resolve the potential dilemma posed in assessing pulses in the extremities with the Doppler principle when more than two limbs are injured. If these maneuvers fail to detect arterial injury, but suspicion persists, angiography is indicated (Figures 9-18–9-21).

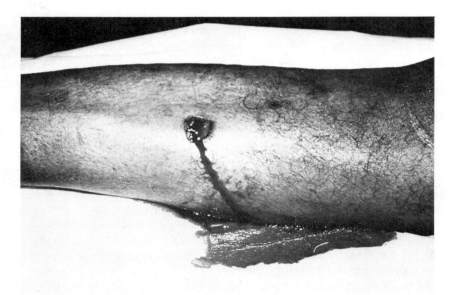

Figure 9-18 A 38-year-old male sustained a civilian gunshot wound of the right leg. The weapon was a 38-caliber handgun. The fired round was a Super Vel type (high-velocity, hollow-nosed, soft-point). No wound of exit exists.

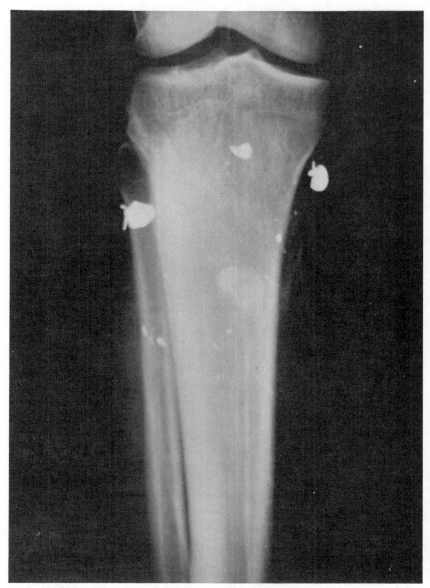

Figure 9-19 Radiographic examination of the leg reveals multiple metallic densities, but no fracture. The patient had no neurovascular symptoms or signs referrable to his right foot and refused hospitalization. He was discharged.

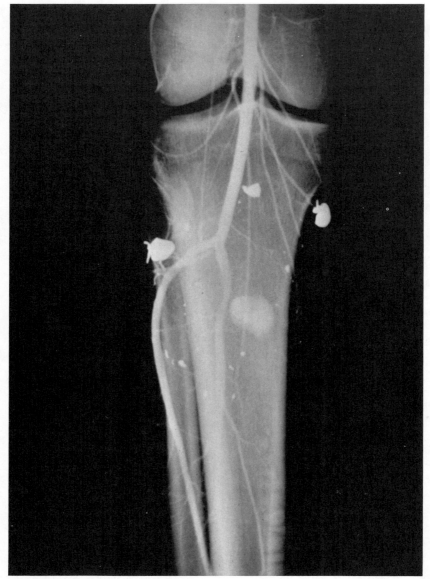

Figure 9-20 Because of persistent right lower extremity pain, the patient sought additional medical advice and was being treated in a "pain clinic" with injections of local anesthesia when a bruit was auscultated over the right knee. Femoral arteriography disclosed a false aneurysm at the origin of the posterior tibial artery with absent filling of the remainder of the artery.

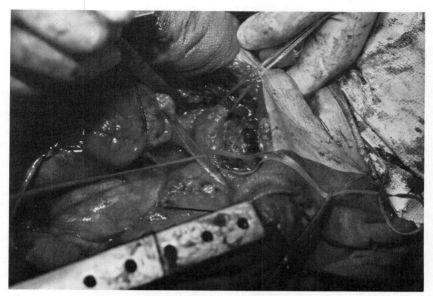

Figure 9-21 The false aneurysm and proximal and distal peroneal artery are encircled with umbilical tapes at surgical exploration of the right lower extremity. The aneurysm was resected and the artery reanastomosed, with relief of symptoms. In this case, the angiogram was indicated by the number and location of the metallic fragments seen on the initial radiogram of the right leg. Surgical exploration would also have been indicated in view of the anatomical probability of one of the branches of the popliteal artery having been injured.

Significant major venous injury is more difficult to detect on initial evaluation. Infrequently major venous injury is heralded by the presence of a clinically detectable hematoma. Nonetheless, such injury must be considered. Distal venous engorgement or measured venous hypertension may indicate venous occlusion by hematoma or thrombosis, or acute arteriovenous fistula. More sophisticated tests such as angiography and plethysmography are available if suspicion persists.

Injury to major nerves within the extremity can be detected through tests of motor or sensory function. Peripheral nerve fields of cutaneous sensation, rather than dermatomal patterns, are of principal interest.

MANAGEMENT

Too few medical professionals and paraprofessionals understand the control of arterial hemorrhage from an injured extremity (see references 18, 19, 20 in Chapter 5). Despite the abundance of training programs within the United States, unnecessary fatal arterial hemorrhage occurs frequently, even after patients have come under professional care. Considering that no vessel outside the trunk is larger in diameter than the index finger, serious or fatal hemorrhage from a vessel of an extremity is inexcusable once the patient is in medical or paramedical hands. Sterile technique is not of pressing concern. Nearly one in ten U.S. servicemen who died in the Korean and Vietnam Wars died from wounds of extremities. This statistic implies that fatal exsanguination was common. All too often, a bulky, absorbent dressing was used rather than the index finger. The use of either a tourniquet or a clamp (Figures 9-22 and 9-23) to control hemorrhage outside the trunk presumes considerable understanding of the consequences. Control of bleeding from a major artery in the field includes, first and foremost, *digital pressure sustained all the way to the operating room.*

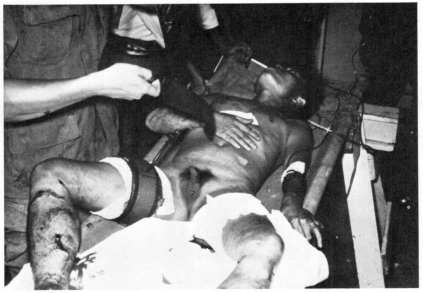

Figure 9-22 A 19-year-old male sustained multiple fragment wounds to his lower extremities from a claymore mine. A pneumatic tourniquet has been immediately applied to his right thigh to control hemorrhage. The left thigh is padded and will be tourniquetted also.

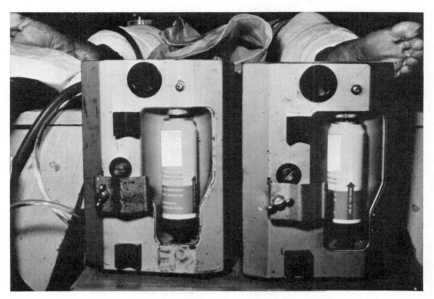

Figure 9-23 The Kidde tourniquet air-source and delivery apparatus are compact and should be available for resuscitation of victims of gunshot wounds of extremities. Pressures of 300 mm Hg and 600 mm Hg are required to control arterial bleeding from upper and lower extremities, respectively. Tourniquet placement can accompany the patient through the radiographic evaluation of his injury, as well as his surgical debridement, if necessary.

A tourniquet (Figures 9-22 and 9-23), whether of the sophisticated pneumatic type used in elective orthopedic and plastic surgery, or the simpler constricting band, is a two-edged sword. When a tourniquet is applied insufficiently tight to arrest arterial flow, but sufficiently tight to arrest venous return, depletion of circulating blood volume results. It is not so widely appreciated that to control bleeding from the lower extremity, a tourniquet pressure of 600 mm Hg usually needs to be applied; and for the upper extremity, 300 mm Hg. The difference between these pressures and arterial systolic pressures reflects the dissipation of force through soft tissue. The pneumatic tourniquet is relatively compact and should lend itself to easy application in the field. Its application is usually painful, unless appropriate padding is used. How long should an arterial tourniquet be applied? *Until more definitive hemostasis can be achieved.* Considering that metabolism in the limb is reduced by one-half to two-thirds for each 10 °C, reduction in temperature in the limb of even a few degrees doubles the permissible duration of stasis of arterial flow by tourniquet.

The MAST (Medical Anti-Shock Trousers) unit is an additional and very useful alternative in the initial management of certain types of major vascular injuries in the lower extremities and pelvis. Primarily designed to restrict blood loss from fractures and venous injuries, as well as literally to autotransfuse trauma victims, it has little application to the control of arterial injuries. An inflatable garment, it compresses the body from ankles to costal margins. Three models are commercially available. MAST I inflates to compress both lower extremities and abdomen simultaneously. MAST II selectively compresses either the lower extremities or the abdomen. MAST III selectively compresses either extremity or the abdomen. These devices must be applied cautiously. Compressing both extremities effects an autotransfusion of approximately two units of whole blood in an adult. Thus, prior to deflation the means must be available for infusion of the same volume of whole blood. Consideration must also be directed to urinary bladder volume, since abdominal compression may damage the bladder if it is not emptied prior to inflation of the unit.

Surgical instruments are useful in controlling hemorrhage from a major vessel of an extremity, but it must be emphasized that these should be vascular instruments (Figure 9-7). Any alternative implies irrevocable crushing damage to the involved vessel. *However well intentioned, application of ordinary surgical clamps will aggravate the vascular injury.*

Arteries

Arterial and venous reconstruction, either primary anastomosis or autologous venous grafting, has in recent decades, primarily through the experience in the Korean and Vietnamese Wars, replaced ligation of major arteries and veins. Three principles in the early management of major vascular trauma resulting from gunshot wounds are the following: (1) when in doubt, explore all wounds of extremities in proximity to major vessels (see Figures 9-1–9-4); (2) repair not only injuries to large arteries (Figures 9-24–9-28), but injuries to large veins as well; and (3) venous reconstruction may be as important to limb salvage as arterial reconstruction when both arterial and venous injury exist (Figures 9-29–9-31).

Angiography is indicated if major arterial injury is otherwise not resolved. Rarely is a false-negative reported with this technique. Angiography can be time consuming depending upon availability of personnel and equipment. If several hours elapse between admission to the resuscitation area and angiography, perhaps it is wise to circumvent the radiographic procedure and proceed directly to the operating room. With one exception the indications for angiography constitute the indications for surgical intervention. Often, the apparent path of the missile suggests the probability of major arterial damage, despite the absence of symptoms, physical signs, and other noninvasive diagnostic signs.

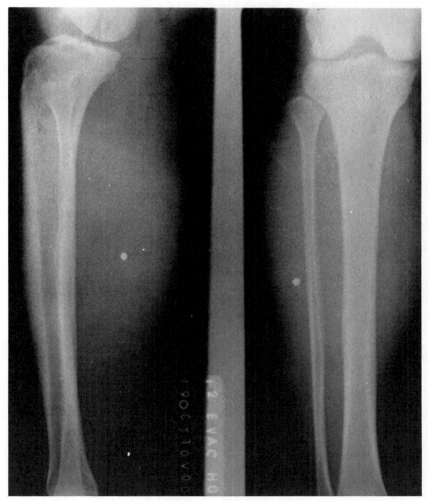

Figure 9-24 Radiographic examinations of the right leg reveal no fracture, but a metallic foreign body characteristic of a claymore-mine pellet.

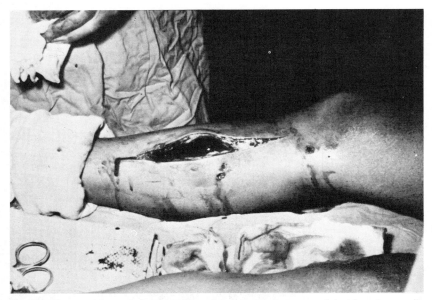

Figure 9-25 The extent of surgical incision necessary to debride adequately this high-velocity missile wound of the right leg is exemplified. Note bulging muscle and hematoma just beneath the fascia.

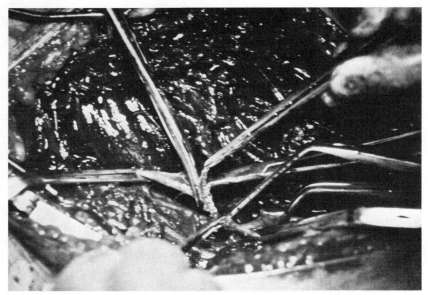

Figure 9-26 Injury to the right superficial femoral artery is controlled proximally and distally, and the vessel is debrided.

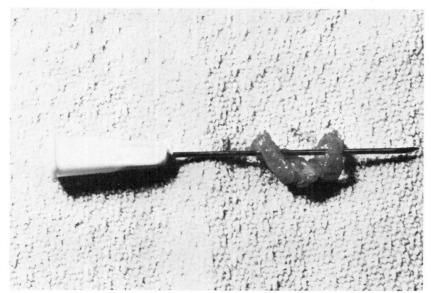

Figure 9-27 The debrided segment is viewed with a #20-gauge needle, indicating the through-and-through nature of the arterial injury.

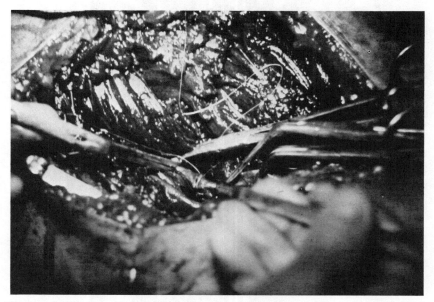

Figure 9-28 Despite excision of a 3-cm segment of the artery, primary anastomosis, the treatment of choice, is made possible by proximal and distal mobilization of the artery and its inherent elastic properties. The repair is performed with 5-0 monofilamentous polyethylene (Prolene).

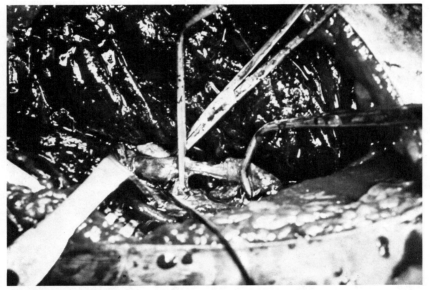

Figure 9-29 More problematic than the arterial injury is the injury to the accompanying right superficial femoral vein. Proximal and distal control have been obtained. Distal venous hypertension (on the left of the figure) is apparent grossly. Because of its larger caliber and less elasticity relative to the artery, considerably greater difficulty is experienced in mobilizing sufficient length for primary anastomosis following debridement, and a suitable autogenous substitute is not readily available. For this reason, ligation or lateral suture technique often accompanied the surgical management of the venous injury when combined arteriovenous injuries resulted from gunshot wounds in the thigh. For reasons discussed, this technique is not recommended.

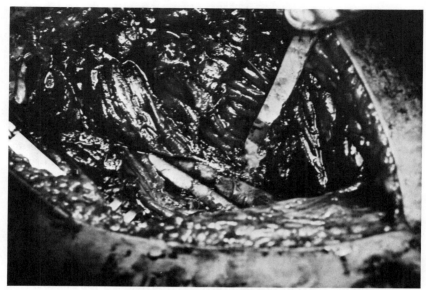

Figure 9-30 Lateral suture technique has been used to repair the superficial femoral vein, and obvious luminal constriction has resulted. The latter obstructs blood flow through the vein and from the limb, but of greater consequence, causes a decrease in flow through the artery and to the limb. This decrease in arterial flow jeopardizes the damaged distal limb, and particularly the arterial reconstruction.

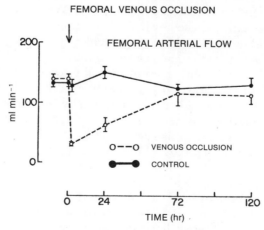

Figure 9-31 An experiment in subhuman primates[29] compares femoral arterial blood flow bilaterally. On one side (o--o), the common femoral vein is ligated (arrow) after control measurements. Flow promptly falls to near zero and does not return to control values until 72 hours later. During this three-day interval, the reduced arterial flow would seriously threaten the success of any arterial reconstruction. Each point on the graph is the mean ± its standard error of five experiments in five monkeys. (Redrawn from: Wright, C.B., and Hobson, R.W. *Surgery* 75:453, 1974.

Assuming that a low-velocity handgun is the wounding agent, and that casualty load is sufficiently high to make triage considerations important, a negative result on angiography could tilt the clinical impression toward a reasonably secure decision to manage the patient nonoperatively, conservatively, or expectantly. This approach would have its obvious advantages in terms of conservation of vital resources, namely, personnel, operating rooms, and associated equipment.

Auscultation over major vessels may be important diagnostically in injuries to extremities. An acute arteriovenous fistula can complicate penetrating trauma to a limb. It requires immediate surgical exploration and repair. Preoperative angiography is desirable. In contrast to the case of chronic A-V fistula, a bruit or a thrill over a major vessel in the injured extremity is relatively rare.

Advances in vascular surgery now enable the surgeon to repair arteries of greater than 2 mm in external diameter without resorting to the operative microscope. Thus, the primary care team should consult a vascular surgeon before indiscriminately ligating such vessels.

Ninety-one percent of major arterial injuries in 1000 cases in the Vietnam War occurred in the extremities.[2] Fifty-seven percent of those 1000 injuries occurred in the lower extremities. The associated amputation rate of 14% was similar to that experienced during the Korean War,[3] (13%) and only a fourth of that witnessed in World War II.[4] Although increasing velocity of missiles and improvements in triage are probably offsetting factors, Rich et al[2] concluded that the difference in amputation rates between World War II and subsequent U.S. wars was mainly caused by the substitution of arterial reconstruction for arterial ligation in the management of arterial injuries. In only 1% of these cases was the major arterial injury treated by ligation.

Popliteal arterial injuries are of special interest. In Rich's[2] series, such injuries were followed by amputation in 30% of cases. In contrast, in a smaller series (275 cases) reported by McNamara, Brief, and Beasley,[5] amputation was necessary in only 12% when both popliteal artery and vein were reconstructed. The difference in amputation rates was significant ($p < 0.01$, chi-square test[6]). Both groups point out that apparent failure to provide for venous drainage contributes to failure of popliteal arterial repair. It is apparent that success of popliteal arterial repair is greatly increased by concomitant repair of the popliteal vein. Rich and McNamara conclude that swelling of the limb secondary to venous ligation causes failure of arterial repair because of a resultant decrease in arterial blood flow and thrombosis at the suture line.

We are often reminded that these reports from surgical experience in the Vietnam War reflect damage caused for the most part by high-velocity missiles from military rifles, mortar, rocket, and artillery, and that such wound management and its predicted outcome find little applicability to the management of civilian trauma in the United States during peacetime. Recent reports cited in earlier chapters suggest that the trend in the United States is away from knives and toward guns as weapons of assault. In a recent report by Hardy, Raju, and Neely, of 360 aortic or arterial injuries,[7] firearms were the offending agent twice as frequently as knives. This appears to be generally true in urban centers in this country today.[8] Current United States civilian injuries reflect gunshot wounds as the etiologic agent in a progressively and surprisingly high incidence when compared to blunt trauma or knife-like instruments. This proportion is almost as high[9] or higher,[10,11] even as high as ten to one[12] in some United States cities. A more recent report supports the continuance of this trend.[13] Thus, the lessons learned from the surgical experience in Vietnam will probably find increasing applicability to the management of civilian trauma in the United States.

Despite the greatly improved prospects for vascular repair, amputation is indicated when other major structures are extensively damaged beyond probable successful repair. In the face of impressive new prospects for arterial repair, the trauma surgeon must not forget the precept of Larrey and Guthrie at Waterloo, recently reiterated by Rich[14] in the context of the Vietnam War, that saving the life takes precedence over saving the limb.

The incidence of amputation following gunshot wounds involving major arteries of the extremity was several times higher during the Vietnam War (13%) than it has been in civilian life in this country (2% to 7%).[15,16] This may be due to the relative severity of the wounds. Remaining unexplained is the discrepancy between these amputation rates for military versus civilian arterial injuries in extremities and associated mortality rates which were 2%[14] and 4% to 12%,[7,8,15-17] respectively.

With this overview of the problem of major vascular injuries in extremities as caused by high-velocity missiles, we now return to more detailed considerations of diagnosis and therapy. We believe that all gunshot wounds in the region of major vessels within an extremity should be explored surgically as a general guideline in the diagnosis, as well as the management, of extremity gunshot wounds (Figures 9-1– 9-7). Negative exploration, while possibly time-consuming, carries a very low morbidity (3%), virtually no mortality,[15] and is often incidental to essential wound debridement.

Snyder et al.[18] analyzed 177 patients with 183 penetrating wounds of the extremity distal to mid-clavicle and inguinal ligament. Eighty-six percent of these patients had been injured by firearms, and all were managed by surgical exploration following angiography. Angiography accurately diagnosed the injury in 92% of the patients. There was no significant morbidity associated with the diagnostic study. Among the

8% of cases in which angiography was inaccurate, there was only one false-negative determination. Angiographic findings regarded as significant by Snyder and associates are evidence of obstruction, extravasation of contrast agent, early venous filling, irregularity of the vessel wall or filling defect, and false aneurysm. The investigators recommend that entrance and exit wounds of the missile be clearly indicated by radiopaque markers. The choice of an arterial injection site should be several centimeters proximal to the suspected injury. Important additional points stressed by these authors include: (1) viewing the vascular tree to the extent of 10 to 15 cm proximal and distal to the suspected site of injury to major vessels; (2) adequate numbers of sequential films for detecting early venous filling; and (3) repeat angiography, perhaps from additional or different viewpoints, if earlier examination yields equivocal results. They recommend that evidence of an intraluminal defect be assumed to represent an injury unless evidence for preexistent disease is strong.

An alternative to radiographic angiography is isotope angiography.[19,20] This technique involves the simple intravenous injection of approximately 1 ml of sodium pertechnetate technetium 99m (12 mCi) and gamma collimation of the isotope distribution apparent in the region of anticipated vascular injury. Utilizing this method in evaluating potential injury to major vessels, Rudavsky[21] reported a false-positive rate of 8% and no false negatives. The accuracy of radiographic or isotopic angiography is impressive. Their use will undoubtedly save many victims of gunshot wounds from unnecessary alternative surgical exploration. However, it is important to understand that when doubt exists, even after angiography, it is safer to explore the suspected vascular injury than to treat expectantly.

If the entrance and exit wounds are not located near the injured vessel, a separate incision for access to the vessel is required. Entrance and exit wounds usually require debridement, of course, but they may not give adequate exposure of the associated injured vessel (Figures 9-5–9-7). Proximal, as well as distal, control of hemorrhage is necessary. Blood vessels, like other structures, require debridement, especially if the wounding agent is a high-velocity missile. Because of their extensibility, arteries can often be debrided and anastomosed primarily. If the arterial injury is too extensive for primary anastomosis an autogenous saphenous vein graft, reversed end-to-end to avoid valvular obstruction, is the best alternative. Major vascular injury should be anticipated in planning the management of wounds of extremities. This includes preparation of a donor site in an uninjured thigh or groin for a saphenous vein, or an upper arm for a brachial vein, graft. Alternatives such as Dacron have been advocated[22] as superior to autogenous vein, but in our opinion, gunshot wounds are usually too contaminated to risk introduction of foreign material in arterial reconstruction. The use of fetal human umbilical vein or bovine artery (heterograft) are probably better than cloth prostheses in vascular reconstruction associated with penetrating trauma, but experience here is limited.

In the lateral suture technique (simple suture closure of the injured vessel with or without debridement, debridement is often inadequate and the lumen is often compromised (Figures 9-29 and 9-30). For these reasons, this technique is not generally recommended. We prefer fine (#5-0), atraumatic monofilamentous, nonabsorbable, polyethylene (Prolene) suture material for reconstructing vessels in extremities. Other nonabsorbable atraumatic suture materials are acceptable, however. Silk and cotton are exceptions because they may break during the late postoperative period.

The question of anticoagulation during extremity vascular repair is moot.[23] Most surgeons, while reluctant to heparinize victims of trauma, advocate anticoagulants when a major artery is clamped. Regional heparinization (5000 units or 50 mg per 500 ml isotonic, 0.9% saline solution instilled into the artery before proximal cross-clamping) resolves this dilemma for some. When treating more distal, and hence smaller, vessels such as the popliteal artery, some have advocated internal shunting, or bypassing the injury[24,25] as is done during carotid arterial surgery. This reduces the chance of distal thrombosis by maintaining arterial inflow to the extremity during repair of the more proximal artery.

Use of the Fogarty catheter to remove a clot distal to an arterial injury has been strongly recommended.[23] Our concern is that too vigorous use of the balloon catheter can cause significant damage to arterial intima, interfere with normally present fibrinolytic mechanisms,[26] and set the stage for thrombosis of the injured vessel. For the same reason that operative anticoagulation is not usually employed, postoperative anticoagulation is rarely indicated in extremity trauma management. The use of antibiotics preoperatively, operatively, or postoperatively, remains debatable. Operative angiography should be performed routinely to ascertain success of arterial repair.[23]

Veins

Surprisingly, the management of venous injury is more complex than the management of arterial trauma because injuries to veins are less evident than those to arteries. In addition, the vein is less extensible and cannot be mobilized as much for primary anastomosis compared to its arterial counterpart, and the larger diameter of veins poses a limit to successful interposition grafting with autogenous vein. For these reasons until recently, injured veins in extremities have usually been ligated.[27]

During the Vietnam War, venous reconstruction was empirically introduced with success. Subsequently, experiments in dogs demonstrated that ligation of a major vein in an extremity causes a profound fall in blood flow through the corresponding artery.[28] When a femoral vein is experimentally ligated in the subhuman primate, femoral arterial flow does not return to control until 72 hours later (Figure 9-14).[29] Presumably this delay reflects the time required for development of collateral venous circulation. While the late sequelae of extremity venous ligation have been well documented, only recently has appreciation of the acute complications appeared in the surgical literature.[27] These complications are: (1) reduced perfusion of the limb can be assumed to impair wound healing; and (2) reduced arterial flow jeopardizes the arterial repair by contributing to thrombosis at the suture lines. Venous reconstruction thus promotes arterial perfusion.

What is an ideal substitute for venous reconstruction in an extremity? The caliber of autogenous vein for grafting in venous reconstruction may be too small under certain circumstances. For example, the diameter of the greater saphenous vein is only a fraction of that of the femoral vein. The internal jugular vein is a possible alternative, but it is not often used to reconstruct injured veins in extremities of trauma victims for obvious reasons. Cloth prostheses, arterial heterograft, and polytetrafluoroethylene are not suitable for venous reconstruction in extremities because of unacceptable thrombosis rates.[30] As mentioned previously, the gunshot wound is considered contaminated and therefore use of such foreign bodies is further contraindicated.

The diameter of the saphenous vein can be effectively increased by compilation grafting (Figure 9-32).[30] In this procedure, each of two segments of saphenous vein of equal length is incised along its longitudinal axis. These two segments are then sutured along their long axes to each other to double luminal diameter. The net result is four suture lines, two longitudinal and two transverse (end-to-end anastomosis). This number of suture lines obviously potentiates venous thrombosis. Even if thrombosis does occur, the benefits of this procedure include: (1) maintenance of arterial inflow at normal levels for the first 24 to 72 hours following arterial reconstruction and thus the enhanced prospects for success of arterial repair; and (2) the fact that thrombosed veins, as opposed to thrombosed arteries, frequently undergo recanalization. The spiral vein graft[31] technique (Figure 9-33) is an alternative to the compilation graft and one which allows for literally any luminal dimension.

What is the relative incidence of pulmonary embolism following venous ligation and venous repair in injuries to the extremities? There is presumably less likelihood of embolization from a ligated vein than from a repaired vein, but this is not reflected by experience in Vietnam,[32] where the incidence of pulmonary embolism was higher in

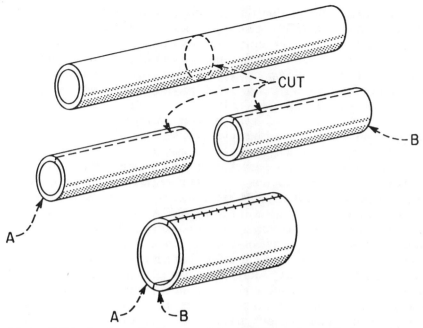

Figure 9-32 A schematic diagram of the technique of compilation grafting in vascular reconstructive surgery.

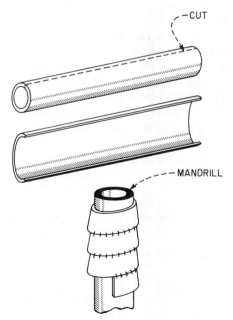

Figure 9-33 A schematic diagram of the spiral vein graft in vascular reconstruction.

patients treated by ligation than in those by venous reconstruction. Our conviction is that reconstruction of major veins injured as a result of gunshot wounds of extremities is mandatory, despite the technical difficulties. We believe this principle is one of the more significant lessons from the Vietnam surgical experience, as significant as the preference for arterial reconstruction over arterial ligation learned in the Korean War and World War II.

Arteriovenous fistulae can develop promptly following penetrating wounds of extremities and may be caused by the missile or secondary missiles such as bony fragments. This complication of vascular trauma should be considered during resuscitation of victims of extremity gunshot wounds. A fistula may be detected clinically by the presence of a thrill on palpation, or a bruit on auscultation of major vessels in the neighborhood of the wound. Angiographic demonstration of an arteriovenous communication is obviously important, since arteriovenous fistulae may compromise circulation during the critical recovery period; may be a nidus for, and source of, bacteremia; and may eventuate in heart failure and unequal limb growth in young patients. The fistula is more easily repaired acutely than after it has become chronic and associated with the development of substantial collateral arterial and venous circulation. Reversal of flow in the artery distal to the fistula and distal venous hypertension[33] are significant additional complications.

Injury to lymphatic vessels in extremities usually poses much less of a problem than it does in injuries to abdomen, chest, and neck. Lacerations of the cisterna chyli, or thoracic duct, must be recognized and the vessel ligated. Someday, perhaps, lymphatic reconstruction may have a role in the surgery of trauma to extremities; at present, ligation is all that is deemed necessary, and development of collateral lymphatic drainage is usually prompt and adequate. A draining lymphatic fistula may result from failure to ligate injured lymphatics, setting the stage for wound infection and threatening nutrition and other major vascular reconstruction.

Nerves

Treatment of injured nerves in wounded extremities remains highly controversial. Previously, such injuries were debrided and reconstruction delayed, since primary repair was rarely successful. Unfortunately, delayed reconstruction is not very successful either. Recent advances in plastic surgery and neurosurgery, including use of the operating microscope and innovative microvascular and peripheral nerve reconstruction techniques such as have been used in reimplantation of extremities following traumatic amputation, may yield better results in the future as discussed in greater detail in Chapter 5.

Bones

Management of fractures of long bones attending gunshot wounds is properly the province of the orthopedic surgeon. As in management of similar wounds of other structures, principles of debridement and secondary reconstruction apply. Conservatism is important, since reconstitution of long-bone defects is fraught with failure. Excision of obviously devitalized tissue is imperative. Every effort should be made to conserve potentially viable tissue. A bone fracture in a gunshot wound is an "open fracture." The chance of infection and osteomyelitis complicating such injuries is thus real. While internal fixation with metallic devices, whether they be intramedullary rods or periosteal plates and screws, has been advocated by some for initial definitive repair of open fractures, most surgeons deplore this practice in a civilian setting because of the high incidence of osteomyelitis. Antibiotics may seem indicated but, there is little evidence verifying their usefulness. We believe that such injuries should be managed by debridement, external metallic fixation,[34] or external immobilization, and delayed reconstruction. Prolonged immobilization and pulmonary embolism usually are not life-threatening in younger individuals likely to be victims of gunshot wounds.

Muscles and Tendons

The question often arises as to whether muscle or tendon should be reconstructed following gunshot wounds. The safest technique is to debride relatively radically and delay reconstruction. When possible, however, and presuming minimal contamination, primary reconstruction is a permissible alternative. Primary skin closure is to be avoided in either case. Determining viability of muscle in wounds of extremities is often difficult. A variety of sophisticated techniques exists. Liquid crystallography, vital staining of tissues, and thermistor probes have all been used to measure muscle temperature. Normal muscle temperature is assumed to indicate adequate circulation and presumed viability. Staining tissues with vital dye relates to integrity of microcirculation and individual cells, but finds more applicability in assessment of thermal injury to skin than in tissue damage secondary to gunshot wounds. The following criteria of viable muscle are useful: color, bleeding on incision, and contractibility to mechanical stimulation, such as a forceps.

In gunshot wounds of skeletal muscle, it is safer to debride to excess than not enough. This principle is confirmed repeatedly by bitter experience. Typically, during the course of a 12-month rotation in a major hospital in Vietnam, the surgeon initially underdebrided. In time and after recognition of the dangers of inadequate debridement he began to achieve the appropriate extent of debridement. To underdebride skeletal muscle is to risk infection by anaerobic bacteria, particularly clostridial organisms. Spreading myositis and loss of limb and even life, may result. Conversely, to overdebride is to risk unnecessary loss of function. Obviously, more objective means of determining the proper extent of debridement are needed, especially for the surgeon who may only occasionally see a gunshot wound.

The demonstration of regeneration of functioning muscle from minced muscle fragments and from autogenous[35,36] free muscle grafts raises hopes that in extensive muscle destruction from gunshot wounds we may someday restore lost motor function rather than accept its loss.

Timely closure of the large wounds which necessarily result following adequate debridement will minimize the cosmetic defect. In delayed primary closure (DPC), experience indicates that the optimal time for closure is five days following the initial debridement (Figures 9-34 and 9-35). Perhaps this interval corresponds to the time associated with maximal mobilization of leukocytes in the wound. Even large, gaping wounds due to a high-velocity missile and the subsequent debridement can be easily reapproximated primarily at five days. Further delay tends to deter reapproximation of tissue and necessitates complicated plastic surgical procedures.

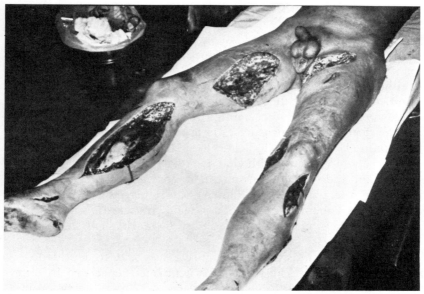

Figure 9-34 Five days following debridement of the extremity wounds, the patient was returned to the operating room.

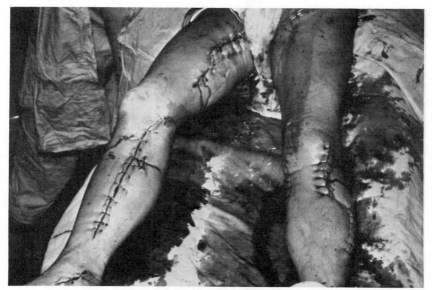

Figure 9-35 Delayed primary closure (DPC) is carried out. Delay in closure much beyond this interval makes closure difficult. Closure earlier than five days risks sepsis.

Application of the foregoing principles to civilian life yields the following results. Recently we reviewed[37] our experience with suspected major vascular injuries (approximately 200 cases) treated over a five-year period (1973 to 1978) at the College Hospital of the College of Medicine and Dentistry of New Jersey in Newark. All patients were victims of trauma. The upper extremity was the site of injury in 27%, the lower extremity in 21% of the cases. Over two-thirds of the patients (69%) sustained arterial injuries. All underwent surgical exploration and this was negative in over a third (39%) of the patients. Although this incidence of negative exploration was high, it was justified in our opinion by the low incidence of complications such as wound infection (15%), mortality (6%), and amputation (0%).

In a consideration of gunshot wounds involving extremities, mention should be made of the problem of bullet embolism.[38] This phenomenon can complicate the diagnosis and therapy of gunshot wounds involving any region of the body, but usually finds expression in the extremities, for obvious reasons. The importance of this relatively rare phenomenon relates to the fact that occasionally, an entrance wound, unaccompanied by an exit wound, remains undiagnosed radiographically regarding precise location of the missile. Despite the usual rule of thumb, namely, radiograph "one body cavity above and one body cavity below" any entrance or exit wound in the A-P and lateral positions, the bullet still may not be seen radiographically.

Total-body radiogram may be necessary to locate the foreign body. Any combination of events is possible. Events range from the "swallowed-bullet syndrome,"[39] in which a maxillofacial gunshot wound results in ingestion of the bullet and its appearance within the gastrointestinal tract, to the converse, namely, a gunshot wound of the abdomen resulting in embolization to a common carotid artery.[40] Awareness of this potential problem may spare the individual responsible for initial management of a victim of a gunshot wound not only the embarrassment relating to incomplete diagnosis, but also valuable time in terms of planned surgical intervention.

SUMMARY

In summary, it is our opinion that in the management of penetrating trauma to extremities the following principles must be followed: (1) careful assessment of the patient to include clinical evaluation of possible peripheral vascular insufficiency by either physical examination, Doppler pulse pressure recording, or angiography; (2) exploration of major vessels when doubt exists; (3) primary repair of both arteries and veins; (4) use of autogenous vein when primary repair is not possible; (5) avoidance of vascular substitutes such as cloth prostheses; (6) general use of broad-spectrum antibiotic coverage preoperatively, operatively, and postoperatively; (7) avoidance of internal fixation of fractures; (8) generous debridement of muscle and other involved tissues; and (9) delayed (five days after debridement) primary closure of wounds.

REFERENCES

1. Tuzzeo, S., Saad, S.A., Hastings, O.M. et al. Management of brachial artery injuries. *Surg Gynecol Obstet.* 146:21–24, 1978.

2. Rich, N.M., Baugh, J.H., and Hughes, C.W. Acute arterial injuries in Vietnam: 1000 cases. *J Trauma.* 10:359–369, 1970.

3. Hughes, C.W. Arterial repair during the Korean War. *Ann Surg.* 147:555–561, 1958.

4. DeBakey, M.E., and Simeone, F.A. Battle injuries of the arteries in World War II: an analysis of 2471 cases. *Ann Surg.* 123:534–579, 1946.

5. McNamara, J.J., Brief, D.K., Beasley, W. et al. Vascular injury in Vietnam combat casualties: results of treatment at the 24th Evacuation Hospital 1 July 1967 to 12 August 1969. *Ann Surg.* 178:143–147, 1973.

6. Snedecor, G.W., and Cochran, W.G. *Statistical Methods.* 6th Ed. Ames, Ia.: University Park Press, 1967.

7. Hardy, J.D., Raju, S., Neely, W.A. et al. Aortic and other arterial injuries. *Ann Surg.* 181:640–653, 1975.

8. Bole, P.V., Purdy, R.T., Munda, R.T. et al. Civilian arterial injuries. *Ann Surg.* 183:13–23, 1976.

9. Josen, A.S., Ferrer, J.M., Forde, K.A. et al. Primary closure of civilian colorectal wounds. *Ann Surg.* 176:782–786, 1972.

10. Steele, M., and Blaisdell, F.W. Treatment of colon injuries. *J Trauma.* 17:557–562, 1977.

11. LoCicero, J., Tajima, T., and Drapanas, T. A half-century of experience in the management of colon injuries: changing concepts. *J Trauma.* 15:575–579, 1975.

12. Mulherin, J.L., and Sawyers, J.L. Evaluation of three methods for managing penetrating colon injuries. *J Trauma.* 15:580–587, 1975.

13. Graham, J.M., Mattox, K.L., Beall, A.C. et al. Traumatic injuries of the inferior vena cava. *Arch Surg.* 113:413–418, 1978.

14. Rich, N.M., Andersen, C.A., Ricotta, J.J. et al. Arterial trauma: A remaining problem of increasing magnitude. *Milit Med.* 142:847–852, 1977.

15. Perry, M.O., Thal, E.R., and Shires, G.T. Management of arterial injuries. *Ann Surg.* 173:403–408, 1971.

16. Drapanas, T., Hewitt, R.L., Weichert, R.F. et al. Civilian vascular injuries: a critical appraisal of three decades of management. *Ann Surg.* 172:351–360, 1970.

17. Lozman, H., Beaufils, A.T., Rossi, G. et al. Vascular trauma observed at an urban hospital center. *Surg Gynecol Obstet.* 146:237–240, 1978.

18. Snyder, W.H., Thal, E.R., Bridges, R.A. et al. The validity of normal arteriography in penetrating trauma. *Arch Surg.* 113:424–428, 1978.

19. Moss, C.M., Rudavsky, A.Z., and Veith, F.J. The value of scinti-angiography in arterial disease. *Arch Surg.* 111:1235–1242, 1976.

20. Moss, C.M., Veith, F.J., Jason, R. et al. Screening isotope angiography in arterial trauma. *Surgery* 86:881–889, 1979.

21. Rudavsky, A.Z. Isotope unmasks arterial injuries in need of repair. *Hosp Tribune.* December, 1978, p. 9.

22. Lau, J.M., Mattox, K.L., Beall, A.C. et al. Use of substitute conduits in traumatic vascular injury. *J Trauma.* 17:541–546, 1977.

23. Snyder, W.H., Watkins, W.L., Whiddon, L.L. et al. Civilian popliteal artery trauma: an 11-year experience with 83 injuries. *Surgery* 85:101–108, 1979.

24. Eger, M., Golcman, L., Goldstein, A. et al. The use of a temporary shunt in the management of arterial vascular injuries. *Surg Gynecol Obstet.* 132:67–70, 1971.

25. Szuchmacher, P.H., and Freed, J.S. Immediate revascularization of the popliteal artery and vein: report of a case. *J Trauma.* 18:142–144, 1978.

26. Malone, J.M., and Gervin, A.S. Letter to the Editor. Embolectomy catheter and endothelial healing. *Surgery* 84:865–866, 1978.

27. Swan, K.G. (Ed.). *Venous Surgery in the Lower Extremities.* St. Louis, Mo.: Warren H. Green, 1975.

28. Wright, C.B., and Swan, K.G. Hemodynamics of venous occlusion in the canine hindlimb. *Surgery* 73:141–146, 1973.

29. Wright, C.B., and Hobson, R.W. Hemodynamic effects of femoral venous occlusion in the subhuman primate. *Surgery* 75:453–460, 1974.

30. Rich, N.M., Hobson, R.W., Wright, C.B. et al. Techniques of venous repair. Edited by K.G. Swan. In *Venous Surgery in the Lower Extremities.* St. Louis, Mo.: Warren H. Green, 1975, pp. 243–256.

31. Chiu, C.J., Terzis, J., and MacRae, M.L. Replacement of superior vena cava with the spiral composite vein graft: a versatile technique. *Ann Thorac Surg.* 17:555–560, 1974.

32. Rich, N.M., Collins, G.J., Andersen, C.A. et al. Autogenous venous interposition grafts in repair of major venous injuries. *J Trauma.* 17:512–520, 1977.

33. Lavigne, J.E., Messina, L.M., Golding, M.R. et al. Fistula size and hemodynamic events within and about canine femoral arteriovenous fistulas. *J Thorac Cardiovasc Surg.* 74:551–556, 1977.

34. Spiegel, P.G. A philosophy of treatment–"The pins that bind us—(and them)." *J Trauma.* (In press) Presented at the 39th Annual Meeting of the American Association for the Surgery of Trauma. Chicago, September 13–15, 1979.

35. Gutman, E., and Hanzlikova, M. Factors affecting success of transplantation in skeletal muscle in the rat. *Recent Adv Myol.* 57–63, 1975.

36. Hall-Craggs, E.C.B., and Brand, P. Effect of previous nerve injury on the regeneration of free autogenous muscle grafts. *Exp Neurol.* 57:275–281, 1977.

37. Report of the Medical Audit Committee. College of Medicine and Dentistry of New Jersey–Harrison S. Martland Hospital, 1978.

38. Taylor, M.T., Schlegel, D.M., and Habeggar, E.D. Bullet embolism. *Am J Surg.* 114:457–460, 1967.

39. Morrow, J.S., Haycock, C.E., Lazaro, E. The "swallowed bullet" syndrome. Case Reports. *J Trauma.* 18:464–466, 1978.

40. Duerr, S., and Cocco, T. Gunshot wound of the abdomen with cerebral embolization. *J Trauma.* 17:155–157, 1977.

10 Summary

Those who cannot remember the past are condemned to repeat it.*

The incidence and severity of gunshot wounds among United States civilians today are increasing at an alarming rate and have already become the most frequent form of penetrating injury. Thus, those responsible for the care of victims of trauma must be increasingly aware of the principles of management of such wounds, particularly when missile velocity is high. Training in management has usually been derived from military experience where missile velocities and numbers of casualties are high. Advances in the management of gunshot missile wounds have come largely during wartime and tend to be forgotten during peacetime.

In the Vietnam War, under conditions of combat, casualty management was more favorable than ever before in war; the killed-in-action/wounded-in-action ratio was 1/6.5. While scarcely comparable,

*Santayana, G. *The Life of Reason*. New York: Collier Books-Macmillan, 1962.

217

this ratio in United States civilian life today is, by an intuitive appraisal, much lower. As in the years following other wars, the hard-won lessons of military surgery are already fading from memory and surgical training programs today place less emphasis on them.

Wound ballistics is essential knowledge in the management of most gunshot wounds. Tissue damage is proportional to the loss of kinetic energy of the missile in tissue. This energy loss and tissue damage increase exponentially with the velocity of the missile. An additional phenomenon is that of cavitation, which causes tissue destruction well beyond the missile path through the tissue. The angle of incidence of the missile upon impact and the density of tissue impacted are also important determinants of tissue damage.

Emergency care of the victim of a gunshot wound requires a team approach which includes physicians, nurses, and paramedical personnel. Priorities include attention to establishment of an airway, control of hemorrhage, maintenance of cardiovascular function, and determination of neurologic status. These priorities should be addressed simultaneously rather than in any given order of preference. Insertion of multiple intravenous lines in upper and lower extremities, a nasogastric tube, and a Foley bladder catheter are essential. Resuscitation should begin with Ringer's lactate solution. Where blood loss is significant, it should be treated with prompt administration of whole blood or its components, using type-specific whole blood when complications of hypovolemia are imminent. Prophylactic antibiotic therapy should begin during resuscitation. A tetanus toxoid booster is indicated. Forensic concerns mandate preservation of clothes detailing probable entrance or exit of gunshot wounds, extracted fragments, or ballistic details obtained historically. After determination of neurologic integrity, all clothing is removed and the patient carefully inspected for additional entrance and exit wounds. Radiograms in the A-P and lateral positions, including one body cavity above and one body cavity below any entrance or exit wound, are indicated.

Gunshot wounds of the head usually require special expertise. In addition, they are more likely to be complicated by secondary missiles of bone and teeth. Metal fragments within the head, on radiographic examination imply depressed skull fracture and, in general, indicate neurosurgical intervention through craniectomy and debridement. Exceptions are fragments deep in the brain and involving such neurosurgically inaccessible areas as the brain stem. Significant maxillofacial injuries will probably require tracheostomy and may necessitate external carotid arterial ligation for control of hemorrhage. Debridement and primary closure are indicated in management of such wounds. Mandibular and maxillary fractures require clinical and radiographic identification and internal fixation. A "blowout" fracture of the orbit must be sought; diplopia is a presenting symptom. Management of orbital gunshot wounds depends upon the vision present in the involved eye. Sympathetic ophthalmia may complicate the injured eye, and if vision is absent, enucleation or evisceration of the injured eye is indicated.

All penetrating wounds of the neck should be explored. Concern for spinal cord injury takes precedence over all other concerns in the management of neck wounds, assuming neither life-threatening hemorrhage nor asphyxiation is imminent. Carotid arterial injuries should be repaired primarily if the patient is neurologically intact, and ligated if not. Injuries to the internal jugular vein can be treated with ligation. Air embolus is a concern. Injuries to the larynx and trachea are treated with primary repair, internal stenting, and tracheostomy if the larynx is involved, or conversion to a tracheostomy if just the trachea is involved. Penetrating injury to the esophagus is the most serious threat to patients with neck wounds, because when such injury goes unrecognized it may lead to fatal mediastinitis, empyema, and septicemia. Treatment consists primarily of drainage; repair is important, but secondary to drainage. Wounds of the neck, as wounds of the face, are meticulously debrided and closed primarily.

While very dangerous, gunshot wounds of the chest respond surprisingly well to nonoperative therapy. Tube thoracostomy effects cure in 85% of such injuries, most of which are pulmonary. In these the lung collapses and continues to bleed. Reexpansion of the lung with tube thoracostomy arrests hemorrhage. Autotransfusion is indicated and ideally suits this injury. The color of blood draining from the chest tube is important. Usually it is dark red and reflects pulmonary parenchymal/arterial bleeding. The indication for tube thoracostomy is observation of decreased breath sounds on auscultation of the chest. Radiographic confirmation is not necessary, but if doubt exists and the patient's condition permits, a lateral decubitus film will be diagnostic. A physician must accompany the victim through this procedure, since the latter's condition may deteriorate unexpectedly. When an associated pneumothorax complicates the chest wound, blood drainage from a tube thoracostomy may be bright red. Otherwise, drainage of bright red blood suggests as a source a thoracic systemic artery on the left side of the heart. Thoracotomy will be required for its control. Other indications for thoractomy include uncontrolled air leak (severe tracheobronchial injury), suspected esophageal injury, suspected injury to heart or great vessels, pericardial tamponade, cardiac arrest, continued bleeding through the chest tube in the few hours following its insertion, and later failure of the chest tube to evacuate sufficiently intrapleural blood or blood clot. Injury to the thoracic esophagus necessitates thoracotomy, repair, drainage, and gastrostomy at the minimum. Injuries to the tracheobronchial tree indicate thoracotomy and repair. Proximal tracheostomy is also indicated. Injuries to the thoracic aorta are rarely treated because of rapidly fatal exsanguination. Injuries to the heart are salvageable when first seen, since fatal injury usually prevents successful patient evacuation. These injuries are treated with thoracotomy, pericardiotomy, and suture closure of the cardiac defect. Careful attention to the position of the coronary arteries is essential in suture repair. Diaphragmatic injury seen at thoracotomy mandates exploratory laparotomy, preferably through a separate incision.

All abdominal gunshot wounds should be evaluated with exploratory laparotomy. Damage to the small bowel is the most common injury and is treated with suture plication or resection. Injury to the stomach is treated similarly. Drainage from a nasogastric tube may be clear in the presence of through-and-through penetration of the stomach by gunshot. Injury to the spleen is treated with splenectomy, and to the gallbladder with cholecystectomy. Hepatic wounds are treated according to the severity of parenchymal damage. Small lacerations may require no more than peritoneal drainage; bleeding lacerations require suture closure and drainage. Larger injuries require debridement and suture ligation of exposed vessels and ducts, or even hepatic lobectomy. Left hepatic lobectomy is relatively simple, whereas right hepatic lobectomy is a formidable procedure. It necessitates thoracotomy in addition to laparotomy. An operative mortality of over 50% can be anticipated if trauma to the liver necessitates resection of its right lobe. If the common bile duct is intact, it should not be drained (T-tube) for the postoperative management of wounds of the liver. Wounds of the duodenum and pancreas are treated according to the degree of organ damage, the degree of intraabdominal contamination and the time interval from wounding to surgery. Thus, if minimal injury is associated with minimal intraperitoneal contamination and is under six hours old, debridement and primary closure should be adequate, as long as pancreatic injury is drained externally. Conversely, if there is extensive damage to pancreas or duodenum associated with significant peritoneal soilage, and the wound is more than six hours old, extensive debridement, tube duodenostomy, serosal patching, duodenal diverticulization, or even the Whipple procedure (radical pancreaticoduodenectomy) may be necessary.

Gunshot wounds of the colon are best managed by resection and double-barreled colostomy with a skin bridge between colostomy and mucus fistula. More conservative procedures include suture plication, resection and end-to-end anastomosis, and exteriorization followed by interiorization or conversion to a colostomy. These more conservative procedures are more applicable to injuries to the right colon than to those involving the left colon. Character and quantity of intraluminal contents, degree of intraperitoneal contamination, and interval between wounding and surgery are important considerations in choosing between conservative and more aggressive treatment of colonic gunshot wounds. When "...the safest method of managing all colon injuries (double-barreled colostomy with skin bridge)..." is employed, the surgeon must be cognizant of the fact that subsequent restoration of bowel continuity is much more difficult than closure of a simple ''loop'' colostomy. Digital examination of the rectum is an essential part of the evaluation of the victim of a gunshot wound, particularly if entrance or exit wounds are located in the trunk or thighs. Blood on the examining finger indicates necessity for sigmoid colostomy, coccygectomy, prophylactic pelvic drainage, and irrigation of rectum from above and below with saline at the time of surgery. Rectal injury is probable even if proctosigmoidoscopy and exploratory laparotomy are negative. Prophylactic pelvic drainage is an adjunct to any colonic injury, since a common complication of such wounds is pelvic abscess.

Gunshot wounds to major blood vessels in the abdomen are difficult problems, since the peritoneum is usually penetrated and tamponade thus unlikely. Thoracic aortic cross-clamping and rapid medial mobilization of the viscera in the left side of the abdomen will assist attempts to control and repair defects in the abdominal aorta and its branches. Injuries to the suprarenal inferior vena cava can be bypassed with a large catheter inserted into the right atrium and secured with ligatures around the suprarenal and supradiaphragmatic inferior vena cava. Lesser, more distal, injuries to either vena cava or aorta can be controlled with partially occluding clamps and lateral suture technique.

Injuries to the iliac vessels in the pelvis are very difficult problems especially when pelvic veins are involved and the pelvic peritoneum is torn. The variety of techniques recommended for control of bleeding from such injuries attests to the disappointing results attending attempts at hemostasis. Suture ligation, packing, embolization, and tributary vascular ligation are some of these techniques. The abdomen is best explored through a long midline incision. Prophylactic antibiotics are probably indicated when bowel perforation is suspected preoperatively. Delayed primary closure of the abdominal incision is wise if intraperitoneal contamination is significant.

Gunshot wounds of the urinary tract almost invariably produce bright red blood in the drainage from a catheter in the bladder. This catheter becomes a useful tool in identifying such injuries and is mandatory in the initial management of gunshot wounds of the trunk and thighs. When gross hematuria is observed, intravenous pyelography is indicated. If this test is negative, cystography should be performed. Cystoscopy is contraindicated. These radiographic tests will usually identify the location of the injury. Bleeding from the urethra demands urethrography. Wounds of the kidney are usually treated with nephrectomy. Attempts at partial nephrectomy are indicated whenever possible to preserve renal function. However, because of associated injuries, the damaged kidney rarely is treated so conservatively. Injuries to the ureter require repair and drainage. Occasionally, renal autotransplantation is indicated when extensive ureteral injury is associated with a normal kidney and bladder. Injuries to the bladder are treated with primary repair utilizing absorbable suture in a two-layer closure over a suprapubic cystostomy catheter. When the bladder injury approaches the trigone, attention to the location of the ureteral orifices assumes importance, and their identification with ureteral catheters is indicated. Injury to the urethra is treated with primary repair and urethral catheterization. Urethral stricture may result, but will usually respond to periodic dilation.

Gunshot wounds to the external genitalia are treated with debridement and primary closure. If orchiectomy is necessary, the hemiscrotum must be drained (Penrose). Abdominal gunshot wounds in the presence of a gravid uterus may require difficult decisions. Maternal survival transcends fetal well-being, since optimal chance for fetal survival depends upon maternal survival. This consideration must enter into preoperative planning. At laparotomy, hysterectomy is indicated if the damaged uterus is beyond repair. If the fetus is near term and viable, cesarean section or hysterectomy may be necessary for more adequate exposure of injury to other abdominal organs. Fetal distress is an additional indication for cesarean section when a gunshot wound threatens pregnancy and the fetus is near term.

The seriousness of gunshot wounds of the extremities depends upon the degree of involvement of major vessels. Fracture of bone is by definition open and thus internal fixation is contraindicated. Debridement and external fixation or immobilization is indicated under such circumstances. Assessment of vascular integrity is necessary. Palpation of a normal distal arterial pulse does not confirm integrity of the proximal artery. Similarly, determination of distal arterial pulse pressure with the Doppler pulse pressure recording device may reveal a normal value despite significant proximal arterial injury. Angiography, whether by radionuclides or radiopaque material, may resolve the dilemma. Where doubt exists, it is safest to explore all penetrating wounds of extremities in the region of major vessels. Arterial injury should be repaired primarily after debridement. End-to-end anastomosis is optimal. The alternative is interposing reversed autologous saphenous vein. A cloth prosthesis is contraindicated, in our opinion. Injuries to veins are difficult problems. Use of autogenous internal jugular vein, compilation grafts, or spiral vein grafting techniques are possible solutions. Ligation is unacceptable because the resulting reduction in arterial inflow to an extremity jeopardizes the viability of the limb. Equally important, venous ligation significantly reduces the chance for successful primary arterial repair when concomitant vascular injuries exist. Debridement and delayed primary closure are the preferred management of wounds of extremities. At present, gunshot wounds of peripheral nerves require identification of the nerve, its debridement, and delayed reconstruction. The same is true for injuries to tendons.

BALLISTICS

Newer types of firearms, readily available for crime and hunting, are achieving muzzle velocities ($> 5{,}000$ ft/sec) several times that of firearms developed earlier in this century. Because of the relation between kinetic energy and velocity of such a missile, coupled with the phenomenon of cavitation in tissue wounds from these missiles, the result will simulate a shark bite, virtually self-debriding, but posing major new challenges to the reconstruction of tissue.

PROTECTIVE GARMENTS

The increasing demand for use of protective garments by law enforcement and military personnel may extend to criminals. Some gunshot wounds that otherwise would have penetrated, may become even more dangerous due to pulmonary and myocardial contusions. Flaunting in the press of the use of such "chest protectors" for VIPs and law enforcement officers will inevitably increase the relative incidence of head and abdominal wounds in such individuals:

The President's Safety

To the Editor:
Law enforcement officers realized some time ago that the phrase, "bullet-proof vest" must be replaced by the current terminology, "protective garment." Likewise, they eliminated use of those vests which could be easily recognized and replaced them with carefully constructed body shields that even light sport clothes could conceal. This was all done for a very specific reason. An adversary who knows in advance, or recognizes on sight, the wearing of body armor by his intended victim, knows he must shoot for the head otherwise the initial shot will not only reveal the assailant's identity, it will also fail to inflict damage.

I was appalled to see on the front page of the Sept. 12 *Times* a description of the President's "protective garment." Of course, the press generally and the major news commentators revealed detailed pictures on television of the President wearing the protective device during his public appearance yesterday. Now all future assassins can more efficiently, and probably productively, plot their course.

Kenneth G. Swan, M.D.
Associate Professor, Surgery
New Jersey Medical School
Newark, Sept. 19, 1975

With regard to protective helmets, U.S. vs German military experience indicates a need to cover the mastoid region to better protect the base of the skull.

RESUSCITATION

Emergency care organizations may take the direction of better design, converting part of the emergency room into an operating room with radiographic capability incorporated into the operating table. Monitoring equipment and type-specific whole blood should be immediately available. Use of these should be supervised by a full-time emergency room physician. Ideally, an anesthesiologist or other individual expert in airway care, should also be immediately available. In the future, we may see emergency care of trauma taking the form of mobile emergency rooms. Operating and radiographic capabilities would be delivered to the vicinity of the injured, with an operating team capable of delivering instantaneous definitive resuscitation. This has already been developed by the military.

HEAD

Better means of extracting missiles from the region of the brain stem, the discovery of principles of repair and regeneration in central neural tissue, and the development of means to control axonal sprouting may, in the future, change the present dismal prospect for such wounds.

NECK

As in other regions, the repair of gunshot wounds of the neck would be greatly facilitated by the availability of better "on the shelf" arterial and venous substitutes. A new and more simply applied principle for safely and reliably immobilizing the head in extension at the scene of the injury would reduce the incidence of cervical spine fracture and resultant iatrogenic spinal cord damage.

CHEST

A simple and reliable method of autotransfusion in chest wounds would substantially reduce the demand for, and dangers of, homologous blood transfusion. "On the shelf" prostheses for large tracheobronchial defects, incorporating a rigid substitute for cartilage, are needed.

ABDOMEN

A better noninvasive radioisotopic test for determining small amounts of blood in the peritoneal cavity is needed. This capability is critical in diagnosing abdominal wounds. Ultrasonography is currently capable of demonstrating as little as 100 ml of intraperitoneal blood. (Goldberg, B.B., Goodman, G.A., and Clearfield, H.R. Evaluation of ascites by ultrasound. *Radiology* 96:15–22, 1970.) It can be expected to come into more general use for evaluating such trauma.

GENITOURINARY TRACT

Some techniques developed for renal transplantation may eventually be applied in repair of gunshot wounds. The organ would be temporarily removed for repair, then reimplanted. Such a technique could someday extend to repair of the heart, larynx, and spleen.

EXTREMITIES

Production of a cone-shaped tourniquet to replace the current cylindrical type is necessary if extremity nerve injury is to be eliminated in using pneumatic tourniquets for arresting hemorrhage from gunshot wounds. Along with better "on the shelf" large vessel prostheses, there will be increasing need, in the face of increasing muzzle velocities, for minces of striated muscle and bone cells. The prospect of extending this technique to the development of autogenous implantation of substitute tissue would substantially improve the prospects for reconstructive surgery after gunshot wounds.

APPENDIX

The following articles and letters to the editor illustrate several tragic cases of preventable exsanguination.

In the first case, a boy bled to death in front of hundreds of onlookers, as the result of an attack by a circus leopard.

Criminal negligence was rejected yesterday by the Morris County Prosecutor's Office in the mauling death of a five-year-old Sussex County boy, who was attacked by a leopard during a benefit circus performance in Washington Township.

Jerome J. Vaccarezza of Byram was attacked at 8:30 p.m. Thursday by the leopard as he returned with a young friend to his seat inside the Roberts Brothers Circus tent at the Flocktown Road School on Schooley's Mountain.

He was taken to Hackettstown Community Hospital, where he died 90 minutes later, according to Police Chief George Kluetz.

"I don't at this time see any criminal prosecution against anyone," Morris County Prosecutor Peter Manahan said. "I don't see that the situation warrants a criminal prosecution."

The child's death was termed "accidental" by Morris County Medical Examiner Kenneth Brinza after an autopsy yesterday afternoon. He said the child suffered large puncture wounds on the back of his neck and died from hemorrhaging and cardiac arrest.

Police said the boy, a son of Mr. and Mrs. Jerome F. Vaccarezza, was taken to the circus by the family's next door neighbors, Edward and Patricia Eyrich, who brought along their 10-year-old daughter, Mary Jo.

Manahan said Jerome and Mary Jo were attacked by the leopard, which was chained to a long leash inside the circus ring, as they returned to the bleachers from a trip to the restrooms in the school.

One of the four firemen serving as guards in the tent, Henry Van Solkema, immediately ran to the children's aid and managed to pull the girl to safety, but could not reach the boy before the leopard grabbed him by the neck and began to drag him, authorities said.

The leopard was one of three cats in an act owned by Conny and Helge Dam of Gibsonton, Fla. The leopards were chained to the ground outside their cages because they were to follow the act in the center ring at the time of the attack, Manahan said.

While a number of the 800 spectators in the tent watched in horror and others ran for help, the ringmaster, identified by police as David Brown, and the animal trainer, Conny Dam, struggled to free the boy.

Brown was mauled on the arm when he attempted to pull the leopard off the boy, while the trainer whipped the animal with a leather strap.

Even after the incident, police allowed the performance to continue to avoid "confusion and panic," Chief Kluetz said.

As authorities yesterday attempted to piece together the tragedy, a number of discrepancies arose in accounts given by officials and some witnesses.

One conflict developed over who authorized the release of the 175-pound, female leopard in its owners' custody. Police said the Dams, who work with the Roberts Bros. on a contractual basis, took their two leopards and a jaguar to Pennsylvania yesterday.

Although Kluetz said conservation officer George Aber of the State Division of Fish, Game and Shellfisheries authorized the cat's release when he arrived on the scene late Thursday night, Aber denied making the decision.

Aber, whose division regulates the treatment and proper exhibition of circus animals in New Jersey said he merely told police the animal's permits were in order.

He added his division and the federal regulating agency, the U.S. Department of Agriculture, are investigating the attack.

Although authorities maintain the audience was warned twice over a public address system to remain seated and away from the animals, Eyrich, the Vaccarezzas' neighbor, said he heard no such warnings and disputed police accounts of other key points.

"I never heard any announcement like that, and neither did the people sitting around us," he said. "The PA system was just terrible; you couldn't hear any words clearly.

"My daughter and J.J. (Jerome) were returning after leaving to go to the bathroom," Eyrich said. "They were holding hands. As they walked past the empty cat cages and headed up the aisle the leopard leaped on them, knocking them both down.

"That chain holding the leopard was about 20 feet long," which Eyrich said indicated the cat's striking range extended outside the ring.

"Those kids never walked up to the cat. They were coming back to their seats," he said. "The cat just jumped off its pedestal and attacked. I raced down the bleachers and at the animal. It had J.J.'s head in its mouth. I tore the cat from him and carried him outside."

The attack occurred shortly after the circus, based in Sarasota, Fla., had begun its second of two performances Thursday night in a benefit sponsored by the Schooley's Mountain Fire Protection Association.

Attorneys for the firefighters yesterday advised them not to discuss the incident, police said.

By yesterday morning, the traveling circus, scheduled for a one-night appearance on Schooley's Mountain, had packed its tents and equipment and moved to its next performance in the Laurence Harbor section of Old Bridge in Middlesex County.

Circus officials declined comment on the mauling.

The Rev. Joseph LoGatto, of St. Michael's Church in Netcong, who administered last rites to the boy in the hospital Thursday night, said the parents have "very good neighbors. They've been very close for many years. The whole neighborhood helps each other, like family."

Father LoGatto said the Vaccarezzas' nine-year-old daughter died of leukemia seven years ago.

Vaccarezza, a biology teacher in Queen of Peace High School, North Arlington, for the past 19 years, and his wife, Joan, have two other children, John and Elaine.

A Mass will be offered at 10 a.m. Monday in St. Michael's Church, Netcong, following the funeral at the Pichi Funeral Home, 105 Main St., Stanhope.

In addition to the immediate family, the boy is survived by his grandparents, Mr. and Mrs. Hector Vaccarezza and Mr. and Mrs. Stephen Keane.

(Gordon, D., and Marks, P. Boy's mauling death at circus ruled "accidental" by lawmen. Newark, N.J.: *The Star-Ledger* 66(102):1, 1979. Reprinted with permission.)

In a subsequent letter to the editor, one of the authors of this text questioned the fact that no one at the scene moved to save the boy.

The fate of a five-year-old Sussex County boy who was attacked by a circus leopard was literally in the hands of hundreds of onlookers attending the performance at the Flocktown Road School on Schooley's Mountain.

He "...suffered large puncture wounds...of his neck and died from hemorrhaging..." according to the county's medical examiner. A large blood vessel was reportedly injured. Accidental death was determined by the county prosecutor.

The unmentioned tragedy is the apparent failure of anyone on the scene to apply basic first aid to the young victim. Presumably, a left carotid artery, or jugular vein, was injured by the leopard. No blood vessel outside of the human trunk (chest and abdomen) is larger in diameter than an adult's index finger, which is thus ideally suited for direct compression of any source of external hemorrhage sustained by a victim of trauma.

Assuming no information to the contrary was withheld from the news report, I would have to conclude that failure by any one of many, presumably trained in first aid, to institute a rather basic technique, direct digital pressure, to J.J. Vaccarezza's neck contributed as much to his demise as the leopard's fangs.

For a five-year-old to bleed to death from an external wound in public is a great tragedy!

Kenneth G. Swan, M.D.,
Professor of Surgery,
Chief, Section of General Surgery,
College Hospital,
College of Medicine and Dentistry of N.J.
Newark

(Newark, N.J.: *The Star-Ledger.*)

The second case involved a schoolgirl who died from head, neck, and chest wounds resulting from shattering glass from a firecracker explosion.

A powerful firecracker exploded in a glass-encased fire extinguisher cabinet yesterday in the Cliffside Park, N.J., High

School, spraying a hallway with glass shards that killed a 14-year-old girl and injured two other students, the police said.

The dead girl, Elizabeth Hennessy, a freshman and honor roll student, had just finished her lunch and was turning a corner toward a first-floor science classroom when the blast shattered the glass door·of the extinguisher case at 12:38 P.M., 20 seconds after the end of the school's sixth period.

The hallway was filled with students walking to their seventh-period classes. The Hennessy girl was said to have been directly in front of the 2½-foot by 1½-foot wall unit. She was struck in the head, neck and chest by the flying glass, suffering deep cuts that set off massive bleeding, authorities said.

The two other students suffered less serious facial and hand cuts, were treated at Englewood Hospital and released. They were identified as Denise Davino, 14, of Cliffside Park, and Anthony Cancian, 16, of Fairview.

Jerry Vella, a science teacher who was near the Hennessy girl, applied pressure to a neck artery at the scene and in an ambulance en route to Englewood Hospital. But the girl died on the hospital operating table.

"She lost a tremendous amount of blood," said Cliffside Park's school superintendent, James Colagreco. "He (Vella) did a commendable job. He saved her all the way to the hospital."

Mr. Colagreco said authorities believed the firecracker— apparently either an "ash can" or "barrel-bomb"—was placed in the extinguisher case moments before students were released from sixth-period classes.

The device was powerful enough to dent the fire extinguisher and the metal back of the case, which was embedded about a foot deep in a concrete wall.

"Whoever did it is living in his own hell tonight," Mr. Colagreco said. "I'm sure we'll find him."

He said there had not been any previous incidents of firecrackers being set in the school of 1,200, situated about two miles south of the George Washington Bridge. "There was no provocation," he said.

(Hanley, R. Firecracker blast in glass case kills a Jersey schoolgirl, 14. *The New York Times*, May 25, 1976. Reprinted with permission.)

The author again wrote a letter to the editor, pointing to the likelihood that onlookers could have prevented the death.

The death of 14-year-old Elizabeth Hennessy (news story, May 25) is a double tragedy reminiscent of an incident two years ago ("A Man's Life," editorial, May 25, 1974). In each case, man's inhumanity to man resulted in a fatal laceration of the victim's neck and, according to the reports, "severing an artery." In the earlier case the patient bled to death on West 32d Street in New York City. In the Hennessy case, since no information to the contrary is provided, the reader must assume that the victim bled to death in the school or else on the way to the hospital.

For a youth to bleed to death in the middle of the day in a public institution is tragic and suggests shortcomings in fundamentals of first-aid instruction, a critical source of man's humanity to his fellow man.

While it is important that we focus attention on the wanton injury, it is equally important that we demand of ourselves an explanation why we permit a group of people to stand around and watch someone bleed to death knowing, as does every good first-aider, that five pounds of pressure on the end of one index finger on the part of one person probably would have saved this girl's life.

The similarity of these two cases suggests that first-aid education among the public is woefully inadequate and that at Federal, state and local levels steps should be initiated to correct this deficiency. Obviously, a good starting place would be the high school. In Elizabeth Hennessy's school, a good place to start would be where she was fatally injured, "in the science wing of the rambling red-brick high school."

KENNETH G. SWAN, M.D.
Director, Div. of General and Vascular
Surgery, New Jersey Medical School
Newark, May, 28, 1976

(*The New York Times,* June 19, 1976. Reprinted with permission.)

In the third incident cited, a man was slashed in an argument over a dog. This man also bled to death as several people stood watching.

Ten years ago, Ronald Sedlock, then 17 years old, came to New York City to study and play football at Columbia University. On Saturday, at 1:30 in the afternoon, he told a man to stop dragging a dog down West 32d Street. The man turned and cut Mr. Sedlock's neck with a straight razor, leaving him dead.

According to detectives of the Third Division Homicide Bureau, Mr. Sedlock was one of a cluster of half a dozen men chatting in the sunshine in front of the Aberdeen Hotel at 17 West 32d Street. Cars were passing by, there were a number of people walking.

A black man, about 35 years old, was reportedly tugging harshly on the leash of a balking dog. Witnesses reported that Mr. Sedlock mentioned to one of the men he was standing with that this was "no way to treat an animal."

The dog's owner, who was accompanied by a woman, overheard the remark and turned, cursing Mr. Sedlock, who, according to the witnesses, repeated his protest.

The police quoted witnesses as having said that the stranger turned quickly with the razor and slashed Mr. Sedlock across the stomach and then across the back of the neck. The attacker, his dog and the woman then ran into the Martinique Hotel, at 32d and Broadway, and fled.

Mr. Sedlock died almost instantly on the sidewalk. An artery had been severed, and he bled so profusely that the first passers-by to call the police assumed that he had fallen or jumped from a high window.

The police have broadcast an alarm for the suspect identifying him as being about 5 feet 9, 170 pounds, medium complexion and short hair. They also have appealed for additional witnesses to come forward.

Yesterday at the Aberdeen, a 200-room hotel, the desk clerk said that Mr. Sedlock had lived there since last July and was a loner. A number of other men said they did not know the victim. One man said he thought Mr. Sedlock had had a drinking problem and "he was working to beat it."

A 1966 roster of Columbia's football team listed Mr. Sedlock as a reserve halfback weighing 175 pounds and standing 5 feet 10. He was a graduate of Shenandoah High School in the hard-coal region of Schuylkill County, Pennsylvania. He had been a star there and had come to Columbia on an athletic scholarship.

Sometime in his junior year, in 1966, Mr. Sedlock suffered a concussion in practice. According to a counselor who knew him, that was followed by a severe personality change. "He was a really nice kid who became confused," said the counselor. "He seemed to have a lot of personalities."

He dropped out of school. At one time he was hospitalized at Bellevue and he became a welfare client. Meanwhile, he made several attempts to return to college, studying anthropology. He was planning to begin again during the coming summer session, according to the detective in charge of the case.

Yesterday, his parents came from Shenandoah to claim the body.

(Kaufman, M.T. Man slain over dog was on Columbia eleven. *The New York Times*, May 20, 1974. Reprinted with permission.)

The author then wrote this letter to the editor, reiterating the tragic lack of assistance from bystanders.

To the Editor:

The real tragedy in the death of Ronald Sedlock ("Man Slain Over Dog," news article May 20) is not so much the fact that he was slain because of his attempt to interdict cruelty to animals or that the assailant was allowed to escape, but rather that apparently no attempt was made to assist the victim.

In the report, Mr. Sedlock is said to have died of wounds of the "stomach" and "back of the neck" and apparently "bled to death" because "an artery had been severed." Had one individual applied his index finger to this damaged vessel with moderate pressure, Mr. Sedlock would in all likelihood be alive today.

At a time when there is extensive utilization of paramedical personnel—emergency medical technicians, corpsmen, policemen, firemen, Boy Scouts, etc.—all with first-aid training, such an incident occurred in the middle of the day, in the middle of a big city, with what was noted as "numerous bystanders." One can only weep at the thought that no such hero could be produced.

Kenneth G. Swan, M.D.
Director, Division of General
and Vascular Surgery
New Jersey Medical School
Newark, May 21, 1974

(*The New York Times*, May 28, 1974. Reprinted with permission.)